PEDIATRIC NURSING

NURSE ● TEST™
A REVIEW SERIES

PEDIATRIC NURSING

Mary Anne Blum Condon, RN,C, MSN
Adelphi University School of Nursing
Garden City, N.Y.;
Former Assistant Professor
College of Nursing
Rutger's University
Newark, N.J.

Series Editor
Laura Gasparis Vonfrolio, RN, MA, CCRN, CEN
Assistant Professor of Nursing
College of Staten Island
Staten Island, N.Y.

Springhouse Corporation
Springhouse, Pennsylvania

Staff

Executive Director, Editorial
Stanley Loeb

Director of Trade and Textbooks
Minnie B. Rose, RN, BSN, MEd

Art Director
John Hubbard

Clinical Consultant
Mary Ann Foley, RN, BSN

Editors
Diane Labus, Kathy Goldberg, Karen L. Zimmermann

Copy Editor
Elizabeth Kiselev

Designers
Stephanie Peters (associate art director), Julie Carleton Barlow,
Don Knauss

Cover Illustration
Marianne Hughes

Manufacturing
Deborah Meiris (manager), Anna Brindisi, T.A. Landis, Jennifer Suter

Contents

Consultant and Contributors

Consultant

Susan L. Jeffries, RN, MSN, Nursing Instructor, Community College of
Allegheny County, Pittsburgh

Contributors

Karlene Albrecht, MA, CCLS, Art Therapist, Johns Hopkins Children's
Center, Baltimore

Nancy Anderson, RN,C, MSN, Nurse-Psychotherapist in Private Practice,
New York

Anne Auerbach, RN,C, BSN, Administrative Director of Nurseries,
Morristown (N.J.) Memorial Hospital

Barbara Biehler, RN, EdD, Assistant Professor of Nursing, University of
Missouri, Columbia

Cecelia A. Boneberg, RN, BA, Nursing Education Training Coordinator
and Medical-Surgical Nurse, U.S. Army, St. Paul

Debra Brewin-Wilson, RN, MSN, CPNP, Editor, Oncology and
Biotechnology News, Plainsboro, N.J.

Christine A. Brosnan, RN,C, MSN, Assistant Professor of Nursing,
Corpus Christi (Tex.) State University

Barbara E. Carey, RN,C, MN, NNP, CCRN, Lecturer, Neonatal Nurse
Practitioner Program, Graduate Division at UCLA; Assistant
Clinical Professor of Pediatrics, University of California, Irvine

Jody L. Church, RN, MN, CPNP, Pediatric Nurse Practitioner, Kaiser
Permanente—Teenage Medicine, Los Angeles

Judith A. Crocco, RN, MSN, Pediatric Clinical Nurse Specialist,
Children's Hospital of New Jersey/United Hospital Medical Center,
Newark

Marie A. Cueman, RN, MSN, Director of Nursing, General Hospital
Center at Passaic (N.J.)

Jane C. Dellert, RN,C, MSN, CPNP, Instructor of Pediatric Nursing, Clara
Maass Medical School of Nursing, Bloomfield, N.J.

Patricia Dillman, RN, MSN, Pediatric Clinical Nurse Specialist,
Children's Hospital of New Jersey/United Hospital Medical Center,
Newark

Patricia A. Edwards, RN,C, MA, Program Director of Graduate Nursing,
Simmons College, Boston

Sandra L. Elvik, RN, MS, CPNP, Medical Coordinator—Family and
Child Advocate Team, Harbor/UCLA Medical Center, Torrance,
Calif.

Karen Kaufman Epstein, RN, BS, MA, Assistant Professor of Nursing,
Orange County Community College, Middletown, N.Y.

Beth Evans, RN, MS, PNP, Pediatric Nurse Practitioner, Fort Worth, Tex.

Naomi R. Fehrle, RN, MSN, CFNP, District Clinical Coordinator, Northwest Health District, Dalton, Ga.

Judy Feret, RN, MS, Pediatric Clinical Nurse Specialist, Pediatric Intensive Care Unit, John Dempsey Hospital—University of Connecticut Health Center, Farmington

Sue Ellen Gaffney, RN, C, MSN, Perinatal Clinical Nurse Specialist and Assistant Clinical Professor, University of Connecticut School of Nursing, Farmington

Beverly P. Giordano, RN, MS, CDE, Endocrinology Clinical Nurse Specialist, The Children's Hospital, Denver

Alice Geraghty Graham, RN, BSN, MA, MS, Assistant Professor of Nursing, College of Staten Island (N.Y.)

Diane M. Hogan, RN, MA, Codirector, Mothertime, Inc., Westfield, N.J.

Hilda Mills Horton, RN, MS, Assistant Professor, Parent-Child Division, Nell Hodgson Woodruff School of Nursing, Emory University, Atlanta

Robbie B. Hughes, RN, EdD, SC, Associate Professor and Head of the Department of Instruction, Clemson (S.C.) University College of Nursing

Debra B. Jones, RN, C, MSN, Perinatal Coordinator of the Allen Pavillion, Columbia-Presbyterian Medical Center, New York

Phyllis Kandl, MA, CCLS, Patient and Family Educator, Comprehensive Hemophilia Center, Saint Michael's Medical Center, Newark, N.J.

Barbara Kellum, RN, MS, Chairperson, Department of Nursing, Orange County Community College, Middletown, N.Y.

Nancy K. Kritzer, RN, BSN, CPN, Coordinator, Case Management Unit—Special Child Health Services, Morristown (N.J.) Memorial Hospital

Dianne C. Kulasa, RN, MSN, Project Coordinator, Prescribed Pediatric Extended Care, The Hattie Larlham Foundation, Mantua, Ohio

Elizabeth Beirne Lade, RN, C, MA, Clinical Nurse Specialist, Morristown (N.J.) Memorial Hospital

Jacqueline Loach, RN, MA, Cardiac Surgery Clinical Nurse Specialist, Charlottesville, Va.

Maureen Matteson-Kane, RN, MSN, Assistant Professor of Nursing, University of Nevada, Las Vegas

Frances M. Melchionne, RN, MA, CDE, Diabetes Clinical Nurse Specialist, Morristown (N.J.) Memorial Hospital

Kim L. Morrissey, RN, MS, Instructor, Rutger's University College of Nursing, Newark, N.J.

Joyce S. Morse, RN, MA, PNP, Former Director of Nursing, Matheny School and Hospital, Peapack, N.J.

Mary Dour Moskowitz, RN, BSN, MS, ACCE, Parent Education Coordinator, The Valley Hospital, Ridgewood, N.J.

Mary E. Muscari, RN, MS, CPNP, Associate Professor of Pediatrics and Psychiatric Nursing, Luzurne County Community College, Nanticoke, Pa.

Susan A. Orshan, RN,C, MA, Doctoral Candidate in Nursing, New York University; Women's Health Care Specialist, Jersey City, N.J.

Judith Page-Lieberman, RN, MS, Assistant Professor of Nursing, William Paterson College of New Jersey, Wayne

Jill Perrone, RN, MSN, Assistant Professor, University of Maine, Orono

Patrice S. Rawlins, RN, MN, Nursing Instructor, Wichita (Kan.) State University

Alice Renick-Ettinger, RN, MSN, CPNP, Project Director, UMDNJ—Robert Wood Johnson University Hospital and Medical School, Department of Pediatrics, New Brunswick, N.J.

Ellen A. Reynolds, RN, MS, Trauma Clinical Nurse Specialist, Children's Hospital of Pittsburgh

Denis F. Riley, RN, BSN, CRTT, Chief of Supplies, Processing, and Distribution, Veterans Administration Medical Center, Orange, N.J.

Tanya M. Sudia Robinson, RN, MN, Faculty, Parent-Child Division, Nell Hodgson Woodruff School of Nursing, Emory University, Atlanta

Deborah DiSchino Ryan, RN, MSN, Assistant Professor of Nursing, Nell Hodgson Woodruff School of Nursing, Emory University, Atlanta

Frances J. Sorge, RN, MS, Associate Professor of Nursing, Niagara University, Niagara Falls, N.Y.

Elizabeth Suraci, RN, MSN, EdM, Doctoral Candidate, Teacher's College, Columbia University, New York

Mary Ellen Symanski, RN, MS, Assistant Professor of Nursing, University of Maine, Orono

Janet L. Thigpen, RN,C, MN, Nursing Director, Special Care Nurseries, Grady Memorial Hospital, Atlanta

Janet P. Tracy, RN, MS, Assistant Professor of Nursing, William Paterson College of New Jersey, Wayne

Laura Gasparis Vonfrolio, RN, MA, CCRN, CEN, Assistant Professor of Nursing, College of Staten Island (N.Y.)

Nona Naegle Wolosin, RN,C, MSN, Family Nurse Practitioner, Blairstown, N.J.

Acknowledgments and Dedication

I would like to extend my appreciation to Craig Blum, PhD, a dear friend, who has taught me how to write and edit; Laura Gasparis Vonfrolio, a friend and educator, who provided me with this opportunity; and my family and friends and all the children I have cared for, as they have taught me much about life and nursing.

To Stefan, John, and William—the joys of my life. And to Clint and Joseph—two of the many children I have cared for and whose presence is etched upon my soul.

Preface

This book is one in a series designed to help nursing students, professional licensed or registered nurses, nurses educated abroad, and nurses returning to the field improve their test-taking skills and increase their theoretical knowledge of nursing. It features case-study situations and a multiple-choice question-and-answer format similar to that used in NCLEX-RN (National Council Licensure Examination for Registered Nurses) and nursing challenge examinations. It also includes a comprehensive examination to test overall knowledge of questions and answers presented in each of the chapters.

Pediatric Nursing offers theoretical and clinical information on the various topics covered in most pediatric nursing textbooks and focuses on:
- understanding children's growth and development
- defining genetic and neonatal concepts
- performing a pediatric assessment
- providing routine well-child care
- handling pediatric emergencies
- treating chronic and acute illnesses
- administering medications and other prescribed treatments
- caring for children with emotional or psychological problems.

When using this book, remember to begin with the first question in each chapter and proceed in a sequential manner. Do not skip around because subsequent questions frequently build on previous ones.

Introduction

Nurses are tested continually throughout their careers—as nursing students in the classroom, as professionals undergoing licensure or certification, and as practicing clinicians in the health care delivery field. Such testing helps to measure acquired knowledge and ultimately prepares nurses for real-life clinical situations.

Because testing knowledge is an important, ongoing aspect of a nurse's career and heavy emphasis is placed upon passing certain critical examinations, such as NCLEX-RN (National Council Licensure Examination for Registered Nurses) and nursing challenge examinations, nurses must rely on practical study guides and effective test-taking strategies if they are to succeed.

NurseTest: A Review Series was developed to help nurses improve their test-taking abilities and increase their general clinical knowledge. Each book in the series focuses on a specific area of study or a speciality of nursing practice. Written in a question-and-answer format, each book includes hundreds of questions built on case-study situations and a final comprehensive examination that tests overall subject knowledge. All questions, which appear at the beginning of each chapter, include four possible answers. The correct answers—along with rationales explaining why the correct answers are appropriate choices and why the incorrect answers are inappropriate—appear at the end of each chapter. A blank answer sheet is provided in each chapter.

Although having a thorough understanding of the clinical material is probably the best way to ensure a good test result, developing and implementing good test-taking strategies may mean the difference between passing and failing. Such strategies include physical and mental preparation, paying attention to directions, keeping track of the time, and reading the questions and answer choices carefully to determine the most appropriate response.

Preparing for the test

Regardless of your reason for taking the test, you'll need to be prepared. If you are like many nurses, this may mean extensive reading, note taking, studying, and reviewing. Therefore, developing good study habits is key. Whether studying alone or in a group, you'll do well to follow a few simple rules:

- Find a place that is conducive to studying, such as a library, study hall, or lounge, if distractions are a problem.
- Limit your studying to several short sessions rather than one long cramming session.
- Highlight only the most essential information, and take selective notes.
- Concentrate on the most difficult or least familiar information first, saving the most familiar information for last.
- Anticipate feeling some anxiety over the test, but try to find ways to relieve it. For example, try practicing deep-breathing exercises and other forms of relaxation, such as rhythmically tensing and relaxing muscle groups throughout your body. Practicing such exercises the

night before the test and even while the papers are being distributed alleviates tension and promotes better concentration.

After what seems like countless hours of studying for an important test, the most effective final preparation is to relax and take it easy. Last-minute cramming can do little to increase knowledge and may cause unneeded stress and fatigue. Exercising or going to a movie the night before the test—then getting a good night's sleep—is usually most helpful.

Taking the test
Before answering any questions, remember to focus on the cardinal rules of test taking:
- Pay attention to directions.
- Read all instructions and questions carefully.
- Answer only what is being asked; do not read into a question anything beyond what is there.
- Know how much time is allotted for the test, and pace yourself accordingly. Be sure to note the halfway time.
- Scan the first page for a question you can answer easily, and mark the answer in the appropriate space on the answer sheet. Then go back to the first question and begin answering the questions in consecutive order. Answering an easy question first may give you a boost of confidence.
- Do not spend excessive time on any one question. If a question seems too difficult or complex, skip the question but remember to circle the number on the answer sheet; then return to the question after completing the other questions.
- Never leave an answer blank or mark two choices for the same answer.
- Compare the test to the answer sheet periodically to ensure that you haven't made any slight but costly errors, such as answering question 4 in question 5's space on the answer sheet.
- Erase all stray marks from the answer sheet before handing in the test.

Choosing the correct response
In a multiple-choice test, determining the correct answer to a question can sometimes be difficult. However, in many cases, you can successfully determine the correct answer by using one or more of the strategies listed below:
- Eliminate any obviously incorrect choices; then, reevaluate the remaining options and choose the most likely response. Ideally, you should try to narrow your choices to two likely candidates, affording yourself a 50% chance of choosing the correct answer. If choosing between the two remaining options seems especially difficult, take an educated guess.
- Look for key words or phrases in the question that can point to a correct response. For example, questions including the words "best," "most appropriate," or "most accurate" usually suggest that the correct response is a true statement,whereas those including "all...except," "least effective," and "least appropriate" usually suggest a false statement as the correct response. Such key words as "immediately,"

"promptly," and "highest priority" usually indicate that the correct response is something a nurse would normally do first.

- Look for interlocking clues, in which the correct response to one question forms the basis of the next question:

---

1 The nurse is caring for Mr. P., who is exhibiting abnormal extension and adduction of the arms, pronation of the wrists, and flexion of the fingers. Which type of posturing is characterized by such abnormalities?
   A. Decorticate
   B. Apraxic
   C. Akinetic
   D. Decerebrate

---

2 The nurse explains to Mr. P.'s daughter that decerebrate posturing typically results from:
   A. Temporary lack of oxygen to the brain
   B. Infection
   C. Brain stem damage
   D. Extrapyramidal system damage

In this example, "decerebrate" (the focus of the second question) is the correct answer to the first question. Although the mere repetition of "decerebrate" might suggest that it is the correct response, the real interlocking clue lies in the logical transition from one question to the other: In this case, the nurse cares for a patient exhibiting abnormal posturing, then explains the nature of such posturing to the patient's daughter.

Important: When looking for interlocking clues, always remember to read the questions and answer choices carefully, as choosing an answer solely on the basis of its repetition in another question can sometimes backfire:

---

1 Which type of posturing is characterized by abnormal flexion and adduction of the arms and by flexion of the fingers and wrists on the chest?
   A. Decorticate
   B. Apraxic
   C. Akinetic
   D. Decerebrate

2 The nurse understands that decerebrate posturing typically results from:

    A. Temporary lack of oxygen to the brain
    B. Infection
    C. Brain stem damage
    D. Extrapyramidal system damage

In this second example, "decerebrate" appears as an answer choice in the first question as well as the focus of the second question. Despite its repetition, however, "decerebrate" is not the correct response to the first question ("decorticate" is correct). The two questions are independent of each other, and no logical transition (or interlocking clue) exists.

After the test
Once you have completed the test, try to put it out of your mind; nothing can change the outcome at this point. Later, however, take time to review the test, if you're given an opportunity to do so—reviewing the questions and answers may provide some insight for future experiences. Otherwise, be satisfied with your accomplishment, and resume your usual work and leisure activities while you wait for the results. And expect to be pleasantly surprised.

Alice Geraghty Graham, RN, BSN, MA, MS
Assistant Professor of Nursing
College of Staten Island
Staten Island, N.Y.

CHAPTER 1

Growth and Development

Questions

1 Which achievement best characterizes the physical development of a 3-month-old infant?

A. A strong Moro reflex
B. A strong tonic-neck reflex
C. The ability to roll over intentionally
D. The ability to lift the head and chest from a prone position

2 Birth weight typically triples by the end of the first:

A. 4 months
B. 6 months
C. 8 months
D. 12 months

3 Which statement best characterizes the normal state of mutuality between an infant and his primary caregiver during the first few months?

A. The caregiver immediately responds to the infant's cries
B. The caregiver understands the infant's distress signals
C. The infant learns that the caregiver will feed him when he is hungry and reposition him when he is restless
D. The caregiver recognizes the infant's signal for restlessness, and the infant quiets when the caregiver repositions him

4 At which age does an infant learn to distinguish himself from his caregivers?

A. 3 months
B. 6 months
C. 9 months
D. 12 months

5 Which behavior indicates that an infant distinguishes himself from his primary caregiver?

A. Smiling at his caregiver
B. Putting his fingers in his caregiver's mouth
C. Crying when his caregiver leaves
D. Crawling away from his caregiver

6 By which age can most children wash their hands and brush their teeth with only minimal supervision?

A. Age 2
B. Age 3
C. Age 6
D. Age 8

7 Which situation best demonstrates the parallel play typical of toddlers?

A. Two toddlers sharing crayons to color separate pictures
B. Two toddlers playing a board game with the play therapist
C. Two toddlers seated next to each other playing with separate dolls
D. A toddler seated on the play therapist's lap playing with a music box

8 Which toy would be most appropriate for a 3-month-old infant?

A. A soft cube with different textures on each side
B. A picture book of baby animals
C. An activity box placed in the infant's crib
D. A set of wooden blocks

9 Which toy would be most appropriate for a 2-year-old child?

A. A bicycle with training wheels
B. A pull toy that makes noise
C. A miniature car or truck
D. A 10-piece wooden puzzle

10 Which question effectively elicits information about a caregiver's knowledge of toilet training?

A. "Have you had any experience with toilet training?"
B. "Has your child shown any interest in toilet training?"
C. "What do you know about toilet training?"
D. "Why do you want to toilet train your child?"

11 All of the following statements about toilet training are true *except:*

A. The child should be given detailed instructions and explanations about elimination
B. Toilet-training sessions should last no longer than 10 minutes
C. Using negative control may hinder toilet training
D. Placing a stool below the toilet serves as a footrest and provides greater stability for the child

12 Which of the following is the normal order of sexual maturity in girls?

A. Appearance of pubic hair, menarche, breast enlargement
B. Menarche, breast enlargement, appearance of pubic hair
C. Breast enlargement, appearance of pubic hair, menarche
D. Appearance of pubic hair, breast enlargement, menarche

13 The first sign of sexual development in boys usually is:

A. Growth of pubic hair
B. Testicular enlargement
C. Nocturnal emissions
D. Deepening voice

14 Piaget's sensorimotor stage is characterized by all of the following *except:*

A. Reflexive behavior
B. Intentional reaching or grasping for an object
C. Habitual, repetitive behavior
D. Regarding inanimate objects as alive

15 Menarche usually occurs:

A. At the onset of puberty
B. In Tanner's stage II
C. In Tanner's stage IV
D. At the onset of senescence

16 Tanner's stage IV of male sexual maturation is characterized by:

A. Increased testicular size
B. Onset of penile growth and pubic hair development
C. Increased genital development and increased growth of pubic and axillary hair
D. Fully mature genitalia and pubic hair *Stage V*

17 Receptive language problems are associated with:

A. Poor grammar
B. Speech pattern or sound alterations
C. Environmental deprivation
D. Problems with decoding information

18 The inability to process symbols and abstract ideas results from:

A. Aphasia
B. Articulation errors
C. Dysfluency *(Speech hesitancy)*
D. Voice rhythm disorder

19 Stuttering is the most common form of:

A. Articulation error
B. Dysfluency
C. Voice disorder
D. Decoding problems

20 All of the following are classic signs of hearing impairment in infants and young children *except:*

A. Unresponsiveness to noise or simple oral commands
B. Gesturing rather than speaking
C. Continuous babbling
D. Avoidance of social interaction

21 Which is the most effective communication aid for a child with a conductive hearing loss?

A. Lip reading
B. Sign language
C. Sign language supplemented by written words
D. A hearing aid

22 Which of the following is the most common cause of inarticulation and poor speech development in children?

A. A hearing deficit
B. A poor role model
C. An unreadiness to develop language skills
D. A palate malformation

SITUATION

Kyle James, age 2, is brought to the well-child clinic by his mother for a routine checkup. After Kyle is weighed and measured by the nurse, he becomes agitated and has a mild temper tantrum. Mrs. James admits that Kyle has frequent tantrums in which he lies on the floor holding his breath and that she typically responds by picking him up because she is afraid he will injure his head.

Questions 23 to 26 refer to this situation.

23 Mrs. James is concerned that Kyle, who weighs 39 lb [18 kg] and measures 35″ [89 cm], has gained only 2 lb (1 kg) and grown 2″ (5 cm) since his 18-month checkup. The nurse responds correctly that based on normal growth patterns, Kyle:

A. Needs to gain more weight because he is not within the normal range
B. Needs to eat more to increase his weight and height to achieve normal levels
C. Is within the normal weight and height range for his age-group
D. Probably will develop an increased appetite during his toddler years, which should help correct any height or weight deficits

24 While assessing Kyle's temper tantrums, the nurse learns from Mrs. James that he sometimes holds his breath until he momentarily faints when he does not get his way. The nurse can differentiate these tantrums from seizures based on the knowledge that:

A. Kyle's episodes usually are provoked by anger
B. Kyle is alert after regaining consciousness
C. Kyle's fainting is caused by holding his breath
D. All of the above

25 The nurse should advise Mrs. James to handle Kyle's temper tantrums by:

A. Ignoring the tantrum
B. Giving in to Kyle's demands
C. Promising Kyle a special surprise if he stops the tantrum
D. Mimicking Kyle's behavior by holding her breath

26 During her assessment, the nurse notes that Kyle responds with "No" whenever he is asked a question. Mrs. James confirms that he acts this way at home, too. The nurse should suggest that Mrs. James handle this problem by:

A. Pretending not to hear Kyle's "No" response
B. Trying to avoid asking Kyle questions
C. Giving Kyle choices and limiting the number of questions
D. Explaining to Kyle why saying "No" is inappropriate

SITUATION

A third-grade teacher consults the school nurse about the growth patterns and general health of two of her 8-year-old students. Andrew, the shortest child in the class, has grown at a rate of 2" (5 cm) per year for the past several years; he has an average-height mother and a tall father, who claims to have always been the shortest of his peers until he spurted after high school. Roberta, who is within the normal height range, has not grown in the previous year; she complains of daily headaches and claims that she cannot see the blackboard.

Questions 27 and 28 refer to this situation.

27 Which condition is the most likely explanation for the short stature of Andrew, who appears to be growing at a normal rate?

A. Genetic or familial shortness
B. Growth hormone deficiency
C. Hypothyroidism
D. Constitutional delay of growth

28 The nurse discovers through a vision screening test that Roberta has complete vision loss in one eye. She determines that, based on the child's signs and symptoms (headaches, vision loss, and poor growth), the appropriate nursing action would be to:

A. Send Roberta's parents a standard form letter notifying them of the vision screening results
B. Recheck Roberta's eyesight and growth in 1 month
C. Call Roberta's pediatrician to discuss the possibility of a brain tumor
D. Request a conference with Roberta's parents and the nursing supervisor to discuss the child's headaches, vision loss, and poor growth

---

SITUATION

Michael, age 13, has been admitted to the pediatric unit for an elective tonsillectomy; this is his first hospitalization. Other than multiple episodes of tonsillitis, he is a healthy and active adolescent. However, he appears apprehensive and has several questions regarding hospital rules.

Questions 29 to 31 refer to this situation.

29 During early adolescence, a child typically:

A. Focuses much attention on body changes
B. Forms close attachments to peers of the opposite sex
C. Begins to develop formal, abstract thinking
D. Develops a sense of community awareness

30 A hospitalized child in the early stage of adolescence may have fears or fantasies about all of the following *except:*

A. Loss of body control
B. Unattractiveness
C. Death
D. Sleepwalking

31 According to Erikson's developmental theory, failure to achieve developmental tasks during adolescence may lead to:

    A. Inferiority
    B. Isolation
    C. Role confusion
    D. Despair

SITUATION

Tyrone, a 15-year-old boy with severe hemophilia A, is admitted to the hospital for the fourth time with a bleeding hip. This time, the bleeding resulted from an injury sustained during a football game, which Tyrone is restricted from playing.

Questions 32 to 34 refer to this situation.

32 Which factor would be *least* important when assigning Tyrone to a room on the unit?

    A. Ensuring Tyrone's privacy
    B. Placing Tyrone with another hemophiliac, regardless of age
    C. Ensuring the opportunity for peer interaction while resting in bed
    D. Ensuring that the room is close to the teenagers' lounge

33 In writing discharge instructions, the nurse reminds Tyrone that he is restricted from playing football. Which form of exercise would be appropriate to recommend?

    A. Swimming
    B. Jogging
    C. Baseball
    D. Racquetball

34 The nurse understands that privacy and confidentiality are important to adolescents and demonstrates this by:

    A. Reassuring Tyrone that his questions and conversations will be kept confidential
    B. Conducting teaching sessions with only his peers in the room
    C. Discussing Tyrone's condition only in front of his parents
    D. Screening all visitors

SITUATION

Cindy, age 8, recently underwent surgery after several days of intensive care and 6 weeks of traction, to correct injuries sustained after being struck by an automobile. She is now in the pediatric unit in a hip spica cast.

Questions 35 to 37 refer to this situation.

35 According to Erikson's developmental theory, school-age children need to develop a sense of mastery over skills. Which nursing action would *not* help to further Cindy's development in this area?

A. Praising Cindy for all appropriate activities
B. Encouraging Cindy to engage in bedside play activities that she can accomplish alone
C. Displaying Cindy's artwork around the unit, even if she denies permission
D. Allowing time for group play and socialization

36 The nurse is aware that Cindy may feel isolated because of her immobility. The best way to encourage Cindy's socialization with her peers is to:

A. Allow her to visit the playroom daily
B. Send any cooperative child from the unit into her room
C. Sit with her for 1 hour each day
D. Install a telephone in her room

37 Which nursing action would be *least* effective in helping Cindy to cope with frequent analgesic injections?

A. Demonstrating injections on a doll
B. Telling Cindy, "This will hurt, but the hurt will go away soon"
C. Allowing Cindy to choose the injection site
D. Administering the injections while Cindy is asleep

SITUATION

Ruth Ann, age 18 months, is admitted to the pediatric unit with bacterial endocarditis. She has a history of a mild seizure disorder and is developmentally disabled by about 6 months. Her anticipated length of stay is 6 weeks, during which time she is scheduled to receive I.V. antibiotic therapy. Her parents plan to visit daily but cannot room-in because they work and have other children at home.

Questions 38 to 40 refer to this situation.

38 Play therapy can be an important part of the treatment plan for Ruth Ann primarily because it:

A. Distracts the child when her parents are unavailable
B. Provides pleasure
C. Helps the child's cognitive, physical, social, and emotional development
D. Helps the child's social and emotional development

39 Which developmental concept is most applicable to an 18-month-old?

A. Separation anxiety
B. Stranger anxiety
C. Egocentricity
D. Distractibility

40 Which play activity would help promote Ruth Ann's cognitive development?

A. Puppetry
B. Pat-a-cake
C. Finger painting
D. Coloring

SITUATION

Martin, age 6, is admitted to the pediatric unit as a newly diagnosed diabetes mellitus patient. He typically cries and has temper tantrums during insulin injections. He refuses to eat at mealtimes.

Questions 41 and 42 refer to this situation.

41 Martin's fear of insulin injections probably results from:

A. Fear of pain and body mutilation
B. Fear of nurses, who are strangers to him
C. Fear that all his blood will leak out of the puncture wound
D. None of the above

42 Which teaching aids are *least* valuable in preparing Martin for medical procedures?

A. Storybooks
B. Videotapes
C. Audiocassette tapes
D. Puppets and dolls

SITUATION

Mr. and Mrs. Stich accompany Billy, age 5, to the pediatric unit, where he is scheduled to undergo a complete medical workup. During the initial interview, the nurse learns that Billy has had three seizures in the past year and that his motor development has been slow. Mr. and Mrs. Stich describe their other children, ages 3 and 8, as normal.

Questions 43 and 44 refer to this situation.

---

43 A collaborative study by several health care professionals reveals that Billy has an I.Q. of 65. Based on this data, the nurse knows that Billy is:

A. Within the lower range of normal intelligence
B. Mildly retarded but educable
C. Moderately retarded but trainable
D. Completely dependent on others for care

---

44 One of the nurse's primary objectives is to:

A. Help Billy's parents gain a realistic concept of his abilities
B. Encourage Billy's parents to persist in helping him to learn something new each day
C. Help Billy's parents to develop a hands-off attitude toward his training
D. Encourage Billy's parents to set lower expectations for him

Answer sheet

	A B C D		A B C D
1	○○○○	31	○○○○
2	○○○○	32	○○○○
3	○○○○	33	○○○○
4	○○○○	34	○○○○
5	○○○○	35	○○○○
6	○○○○	36	○○○○
7	○○○○	37	○○○○
8	○○○○	38	○○○○
9	○○○○	39	○○○○
10	○○○○	40	○○○○
11	○○○○	41	○○○○
12	○○○○	42	○○○○
13	○○○○	43	○○○○
14	○○○○	44	○○○○
15	○○○○		
16	○○○○		
17	○○○○		
18	○○○○		
19	○○○○		
20	○○○○		
21	○○○○		
22	○○○○		
23	○○○○		
24	○○○○		
25	○○○○		
26	○○○○		
27	○○○○		
28	○○○○		
29	○○○○		
30	○○○○		

Answers and rationales

1 Correct answer—**D**

Infant developmental milestones, generally grouped in 3-month increments, include the gain or loss of certain reflexes and the mastery of increasingly sophisticated motor skills. The ability to lift the head and chest from a prone position is characteristic of a 3-month-old infant and demonstrates the cephalocaudal principle of growth and development—that is, the infant's ability to raise his head, then his chest, and then his trunk. The Moro and tonic-neck reflexes usually begin fading at 3 months; a persistently strong Moro or tonic-neck reflex is abnormal. Rolling over also occurs incrementally: The infant begins by rolling from back to side, then from side to back, and then over completely. Rolling over intentionally usually occurs at ages 5 to 6 months.

2 Correct answer—**D**

Birth weight typically doubles by 6 months, triples by 12 months, and quadruples by 30 months.

3 Correct answer—**D**

All of these statements demonstrate positive development in the infant-caregiver relationship, but only the last one exemplifies the concept of mutuality: the special sensing—mutual exchange of unique cues and responses—between an infant and his caregiver that cannot be replicated with a substitute caregiver, such as a nurse. For mutuality to occur, the caregiver must think of the infant as an active participant in the relationship, not as a passive vessel.

4 Correct answer—**C**

Individuation—the process whereby an infant realizes he is a distinct individual with a will of his own—usually occurs at age 8 or 9 months, after the infant has established a trusting relationship with his caregivers. This realization appears to be related to cognitive development.

5 Correct answer—**C**

Stranger anxiety (also called 8-month anxiety) is the most important criterion in determining an infant's ability to distinguish himself from his primary caregiver. Typically, the infant experiencing this type of anxiety cries when the caregiver leaves or a stranger approaches. This behavior usually dissipates by the end of the first year but reappears to a stronger degree at 18 months.

6 Correct answer—**B**

Between ages 2 and 3, most children undergo significant changes in the development of fine motor skills. According to studies based on results of the Denver Developmental Screening Test (DDST), approximately 90% of U.S. children are capable of washing their hands and brushing their teeth with minimal supervision by age 3.

7 Correct answer—**C**

Parallel play refers to noninteractive, side-by-side play in which toddlers engage, as exemplified by two toddlers seated next to each other playing with separate dolls. The situations involving two toddlers sharing crayons or playing a board game do not demonstrate this behavior because toddlers typically do not share and cooperate and because such activity connotes interaction. Also, in the case of two toddlers playing a board game with the play therapist, the play involves interaction with an adult. The situation involving a toddler playing with a music box while seated on the play therapist's lap also does not demonstrate parallel play because the play involves only one toddler, who is interacting with an adult.

8 Correct answer—**A**

A young infant enjoys feeling various textures and is capable of holding a lightweight object, such as a soft cube. A book would hold little interest for an infant so young. An activity box and wooden blocks are too sophisticated for a 3-month-old infant, who has not yet developed the fine and gross motor skills needed for reaching, holding, pulling, and stacking.

9 Correct answer—**B**

Toddlers expend most of their energy walking and enjoy pulling things behind them. A 2-year-old child lacks the gross motor skills necessary to ride a bicycle. Miniature cars require fine motor coordination and are more appropriate for a preschooler. A 10-piece puzzle requires fine motor coordination and higher cognitive development and is therefore too complex for a 2-year-old child.

10 Correct answer—C

The initial step in health education involves assessing an individual's needs, motivation, developmental level, knowledge base, and learning ability. By asking such open-ended questions as, "What do you know about toilet training?" the nurse can elicit information and provide a basis for more specific questions that can lead to teaching. Questions involving the caregiver's previous experience and motivation and the child's readiness for toilet training should be part of the assessment phase, but these questions are too specific to be of value initially.

11 Correct answer—A

Toddlers require simple, clear, and nondetailed instructions and explanations to complete a task. Toilet-training sessions should last no longer than 10 minutes because the toddler's attention span typically ranges from 5 to 10 minutes. Praise for cooperation or successful elimination is more effective than using negative control, such as spanking, which may hinder toilet-training efforts. A stool placed below the toilet can serve as a footrest, providing greater stability and a sense of security for the child.

12 Correct answer—C

Although individuals mature sexually at different rates, most follow a normal developmental rhythm and order. The typical order of female sexual maturity—breast enlargement, followed by appearance of pubic hair, and, finally, menarche—commonly occurs between ages 9 and 17.

13 Correct answer—B

Male sexual development commonly occurs between ages 10 and 17, characteristically beginning with testicular enlargement and scrotal skin reddening. Pubic hair development, nocturnal emissions, and deepening voice—the most notable changes during adolescence—typically follow.

14 Correct answer—D

Regarding inanimate objects as alive (animism) is characteristic of Piaget's preoperational stage of cognitive development, which occurs between ages 2 and 7. Reflexive behavior, intentional reaching or grasping, and habitual, repetitive behavior are characteristic of the sensorimotor stage, which occurs from birth to about age 2.

15 Correct answer—C

Menarche usually occurs in Tanner's stage IV, a latent stage of puberty, characterized in girls by protrusion of the areola and nipple, presence of axillary hair, growth of pubic hair, and beginning of menses (menarche). It does not occur at the onset of puberty or senescence, the stage associated with old age. Tanner's stage II, the stage of early puberty, is marked by the beginning development of secondary sex characteristics, such as breast buds and early pubic hair.

16 Correct answer—C

Tanner's stage IV is characterized in boys by increased genital development, thicker and coarser pubic hair, and increased axillary hair. Stage II is characterized by increased testicular size, as noted by an increased pendulous appearance of the scrotum and the onset of penile growth and pubic hair development. Stage V is marked by fully mature genitalia and pubic hair.

17 Correct answer—D

A child with a receptive language problem has trouble decoding information because he does not understand verbal symbols. He also may have limited comprehension and ability to organize ideas. Poor grammar, speech pattern and sound alterations, and environmental deprivation are associated with expressive speech difficulties.

18 Correct answer—A

The inability to process symbols and abstract ideas usually results from aphasia, a central nervous system dysfunction commonly caused by trauma or inadequate language development. Expressive language problems, such as articulation defects, dysfluency (speech hesitancy), and voice disorders, are symptoms of aphasia.

19 Correct answer—B

Stuttering is the most common form of dysfluency (speech hesitancy), a normal characteristic of speech development during the preschool years. More common in boys, stuttering typically occurs because the child's vocabulary does not keep pace with his advancing mental ability and comprehension level. In many cases, a child under age 3 is unaware that he is stuttering. Stuttering that persists beyond age 5 usually requires caregiver assistance, such as reinforcement of fluent speech periods that occur with singing or repeating nursery rhymes. With proper attention, dysfluency can be reversed early in the child's development. An articulation error involves the incorrect pronunciation of a sound or the omission of a sound, particularly at the end of a word. A voice disorder involves a deviation in the pitch, loudness, or quality of speech. A decoding problem involves difficulty processing and interpreting information in the brain.

20 Correct answer—C

Continuous babbling is not an indication of hearing impairment in an infant or a young child. Hearing impairment usually becomes noticeable when the child exhibits a problem in one or more of the following areas: orientation responses (such as unresponsiveness to simple oral commands), vocalization and sound production (such as absence of babbling or vocal play by age 7 months), visual attentiveness (such as gesturing rather than speaking), socialization and adaptation (such as avoidance of social interaction), and emotional behaviors (such as frequent stubbornness or inattentiveness).

21 Correct answer—D

Conductive hearing loss results from interference of sound transmission to the middle ear. Commonly, this type of hearing loss involves interference with the loudness or volume of sound; therefore, the most effective communication aid for a child with a conductive hearing loss is a hearing aid, which amplifies sound. Lip reading is not as effective as a hearing aid because only about 40% of the spoken word is understood using this technique. Although sign language, a form of visual-gestural communication, is a useful nonverbal tool, it causes the hearing-impaired individual to be more dependent on others for communication and is not as effective as amplification of sound received in the middle ear.

22 Correct answer—A

A hearing deficit is the most common cause of inarticulation and poor speech development in children. A poor role model, the child's unreadiness to develop language skills, and palate malformation also affect inarticulation and poor speech; however, they usually are not the primary cause.

23 Correct answer—C

Growth, which slows considerably during the toddler years, usually occurs in spurts followed by plateaus. A toddler typically gains 4 to 6 lb (1.8 to 2.7 kg) and grows about 3″ (7.6 cm) per year. In this situation, Kyle is within the normal weight and height range for his age-group. He does not need to gain more weight, nor does he need to eat more. Because of the normal decreased rate of growth, his caloric requirements and protein and fluid intake will be lower and his appetite probably will decrease.

24 Correct answer—D

Temper tantrums usually are provoked by anger, frustration, or exhaustion or by an unmet or unrealistic request; seizures are unprovoked. After a temper tantrum, the child is alert and responsive and remembers what happened; after a seizure, the child typically sleeps for a few hours and may awaken with a headache and no memory of the event. During a temper tantrum, the child may faint from lack of oxygen caused by holding his breath; during the tonic stages of a seizure, the child typically falls, then faints from lack of oxygen caused by involuntary respiratory muscle contraction.

25 Correct answer—A

Temper tantrums are a normal part of the psychosocial development of a toddler, who is independent enough to know what he wants but lacks the vocabulary or cognitive skills to express himself in a more socially acceptable way. Tantrums commonly occur when a caregiver makes an unrealistic request or when a child is tired or has difficulty making decisions. As long as the child is not injuring himself, the best way for a caregiver to handle a tantrum is to express disapproval of the behavior, then ignore the tantrum. When the tantrum is over, the caregiver should treat the child warmly, as if nothing happened. Immediately giving in to the child's request may encourage further tantrums. Promising the child a special surprise if he stops the tantrum is a form of bribery and should be discouraged. Mimicking the child's behavior is nontherapeutic and should be discouraged.

26 Correct answer—**C**

Negativism, a normal part of a child's psychosocial development, is the means by which a toddler attempts to control his environment. An effective way of coping with a child who always responds to questions by saying "No" is to give the child choices and limit the number of questions. For example, the caregiver might say, "You can have peanut butter crackers or a tuna fish sandwich for lunch today," which gives the child a choice and avoids posing a question. Ignoring the child's negativism does not allow the caregiver to set limits or help the child to learn self-discipline. Trying to avoid asking the child questions is unrealistic. Explaining in detail that saying "No" is not always appropriate is unrealistic because of the toddler's cognitive level and limited attention span.

27 Correct answer—**D**

Constitutional delay of growth is the most common cause of short stature in a child. Sometimes labeled a "late bloomer," a child with this condition typically grows at a normal rate (about 2″ [5 cm] per year) but enters puberty and achieves adult height later than an average child. Many children with constitutional delay have family members with similar growth patterns. Children with genetic or familial shortness usually have at least one short parent; in this situation, Andrew's parents are average to tall. Children with untreated growth hormone deficiency or hypothyroidism do not grow at a normal rate.

28 Correct answer—**D**

The appropriate nursing action in this case would be to request a conference with Roberta's parents and the nursing supervisor to discuss the child's headaches, vision loss, and poor growth and the need for follow-up evaluation. Sending the parents a standard form letter notifying them of the vision screening results would not guarantee immediate follow-up. Rechecking the child's vision and growth in 1 month without taking immediate action would be inappropriate because vision loss is a serious symptom that warrants a thorough and immediate medical examination. Calling the pediatrician before consulting the parents might be a violation of the child's and parents' confidentiality.

29 Correct answer—A

During early adolescence, a child undergoes tremendous hormonal changes (puberty), resulting in rapid growth and development. This coincides with the child's growing self-awareness, which enables him to focus attention on body image changes. A child usually does not develop close attachments to peers of the opposite sex until midadolescence, when he also begins developing formal, abstract thinking. A child usually does not develop a sense of community awareness until later in adolescence.

30 Correct answer—D

Sleepwalking is a sleep disorder of middle childhood characterized by nonpurposeful nocturnal walking and hand movements; it is uncommon after age 12. During early adolescence, which is typically an intensely emotional period, a child has concerns and fantasies about his body image and social acceptance. Hospitalization may foster fears and fantasies about loss of body control, unattractiveness, and death because it interferes with the adolescent's independence, separates him from his family, and places him in an environment frequently associated with illness, disfigurement, and death.

31 Correct answer—C

According to Erikson's developmental theory, a child should develop ego identity during adolescence. To do so, he must reconcile with the past, separate from his caregivers, incorporate the future, and develop peer and societal relationships. Failure to achieve these tasks results in role confusion, a state in which the adolescent does not know who he is or how or where he fits in. Also according to this theory, failure to achieve industry during middle childhood results in inferiority; failure to achieve intimacy during young adulthood results in isolation; and failure to achieve integrity during later adulthood results in despair.

32 Correct answer—B

An adolescent thrives on interaction with peers who are near his own cognitive level; therefore, the nurse should consider the age of a prospective roommate when assigning Tyrone a room on the unit. Ensuring privacy should be a primary concern regardless of room assignment. This can be accomplished by using curtains and drapes and speaking at an appropriate voice level when discussing Tyrone's condition and treatment. Because hip immobilization is crucial to helping this child recover, the nurse should make every effort to ensure the opportunity for peer interaction while Tyrone rests in bed. The nurse should encourage visits from family, friends, and other teenagers on the unit. Because Tyrone's friends may be unable to visit during normal visiting hours or may have difficulty finding transportation to the hospital, asssigning him a room near the teenagers' lounge maximizes the potential for peer interaction.

33 Correct answer—A

The most appropriate sport to recommend is swimming, which provides excellent muscular strengthening and cardiovascular conditioning. Jogging, baseball, and racquetball should not be recommended because of the danger of head or joint injuries.

34 Correct answer—A

Privacy and confidentiality are important to adolescents. The nurse can best demonstrate an understanding of Tyrone's needs by reassuring him that all questions and conversations will be kept confidential. Adhering to this policy helps to establish a trusting nurse-patient relationship and encourages Tyrone to speak openly. Conducting teaching sessions with others in the room, discussing private issues in front of Tyrone's parents, and screening all visitors may be perceived as an invasion of privacy and could thwart the nurse-patient relationship.

35 Correct answer—C

According to Erikson's theory, failure of a school-age child to develop a sense of mastery over skills can lead to feelings of inferiority. Displaying Cindy's artwork around the unit without her permission may foster such feelings, especially if she does not feel that her work is worthy of display. Praising Cindy for appropriate activities, encouraging individual accomplishment through bedside play activities, and allowing time for group play and socialization are appropriate ways of promoting the development of mastery of skills.

36 Correct answer—A

School-age children need peer interaction and thrive on peer approval and acceptance. Such socialization is difficult in a hospital setting, especially when a child is immobile. Allowing Cindy to visit the playroom on a daily basis provides a nonthreatening environment for peer interaction and helps her to feel less isolated. Sending any cooperative child to visit Cindy would be appropriate only if the child is in the same age-group. Sitting with Cindy for 1 hour each day would not foster the necessary peer interaction or relieve her feelings of isolation. Installing a telephone in Cindy's room would allow her to communicate with family and friends but also could reinforce feelings of physical isolation.

37 Correct answer—D

The nurse should always wake a child before administering an injection; failure to do so may encourage the child's belief that she has no control over the situation, which, according to Erikson, could lead to psychosocial problems in a child. Demonstrating injections on a doll acquaints Cindy with the use of needles and the injection procedure and provides an appropriate outlet for her fears. Telling her that the needle will hurt but that the hurt will go away acknowledges the pain associated with injections and allows her to express fear. Permitting Cindy to choose the injection site, when possible, gives her a sense of control over the situation.

38 Correct answer—C

Theorists commonly refer to play as a child's work and her response to life. It provides the child with a link to the world around her—an essential link if the child is to become a vital and creative adult. Studies have shown that children deprived of adequate opportunities to play and explore their environment sometimes have difficulties in various developmental areas. Play therapy, therefore, would be an important part of the treatment plan, primarily because it enables Ruth Ann to develop cognitively, physically, socially, and emotionally. Play also provides distraction and pleasure; however, they are not the primary purpose of play in this situation.

39 Correct answer—A

According to Anne Freud, a child between ages 8 and 24 months is in the ego-psychological stage of development, during which time she typically is reluctant to separate from her caregiver (separation anxiety). At this time, she also may begin to substitute transitional objects, such as a security blanket or a stuffed animal, for her caregiver. Stranger anxiety, which commonly is manifested by the child's crying when a stranger approaches, usually begins between ages 6 and 8 months. Egocentricity, the ability to view the world from only the child's perspective, is characteristic of Piaget's preoperational stage and occurs between ages 2 and 6. Distractibility is not a developmental concept.

40 Correct answer—B

Playing pat-a-cake helps promote imitation and movement, which are characteristic of Piaget's schematic stage of development that is typical of the 1- to 3-year-old child. Puppetry, which requires imaginative play, is more appropriate for a child ages 2 to 6. Finger painting and coloring require the cognitive skill and physical development that a child achieves between ages 2 and 4.

41 Correct answer—A

Fear of pain and body mutilation are characteristic of Piaget's operational stage of development, which occurs between ages 6 and 12. Fear of strangers is characteristic of 8- to 18-month-old children. A child's fear that all his blood will leak out of the puncture wound is characteristic of a preschooler, whose concept of body integrity is poorly developed.

42 Correct answer—C

Audiocassette tapes would be least valuable in this situation because a typical 6-year-old child thrives on active games and drawing or coloring; listening to a cassette tape would be too passive an activity. Visual and manipulative play materials, such as storybooks, videotapes, and puppets and dolls, are more appropriate for a child of this age.

43 Correct answer—B

According to the American Association on Mental Deficiency, persons with an I.Q. between 50 and 70 are classified as mildly mentally retarded but educable; those with an I.Q. between 36 and 50, moderately mentally retarded but trainable; and those with an I.Q. below 36, severely and profoundly impaired, requiring constant custodial care.

44 Correct answer—A

One of the nurse's main objectives is to help the family of a disabled child accept the child's condition and gain a realistic concept of his abilities. The nurse should encourage the family members to act as the child's primary rehabilitators, treating the effects of the condition rather than the disorder itself. Normalization and mainstreaming are two approaches used to assist mentally retarded children and their families in setting and attaining realistic goals. Another objective is to help the family recognize the need to remain intact and functioning throughout the child's life. The nurse should keep in mind, however, that families adjust to and cope with disability individually and do not necessarily follow a predictable time frame or pattern.

In this situation, Billy's parents should be encouraged to assess his readiness and ability to learn on a daily basis and avoid rigid schedules for learning new tasks or activities. Progress toward goals may be slow and unpredictable; intensive schedules and unrealistic goals may set the child up for failure and lead to a sense of frustration for both the parents and child. Billy's parents also should be encouraged to take an active role in his care and training. Parental reactions to a child with a disability often include rejection, ambivalence, and denial; engaging the parents in the child's care fosters acceptance of the child and his disability. Setting lower expectations for Billy may lower his self-esteem and therefore should be discouraged.

CHAPTER 2

Genetic and Neonatal Concepts

Questions

1 Which term describes the cellular material that carries the genetic code?

A. Deoxyribonucleic acid (DNA)
B. Chromosome
C. Barr body
D. Autosome

2 A normal female karyotype is abbreviated as:

A. 46XY
B. 46XX
C. 47XY
D. 45XX

3 Mr. and Mrs. Davis have a child with a homozygous recessive trait; they are unaffected themselves. The probability of having a second child with the same trait is:

A. 25%
B. 50%
C. 75%
D. 100%

4 Which statement about autosomal dominant inheritance patterns is *true?*

A. Affected persons have unaffected parents who are heterozygous for the trait
B. Family histories are negative for the trait
C. Males are affected exclusively
D. Affected persons always have an affected parent

5 Hemophilia is an X-linked (sex-linked) recessive trait. In this form of inheritance:

A. Males and females are affected equally
B. All sons of an affected male are affected
C. Only daughters of an affected male are affected
D. Daughters of an affected male are carriers

6 When diagnosed early, phenylketonuria can be controlled by:

A. Insulin
B. Pancreatin
C. Braces
D. Diet   *Breast milk*

7 The phenotypic features of epicanthal folds, simian creases, hypotonia, flat nasal bridge, and tongue protrusion are associated with:

A. Trisomy 13
B. Trisomy 18
C. Trisomy 21
D. Trisomy 46

8 Twins that share the same specific traits are called:

A. Discordant
B. Concordant
C. Dizygotic
D. Fraternal

9 To obtain an accurate rectal temperature in a neonate, the nurse should insert the thermometer:

A. ¼″ (about 0.5 cm)
B. ½″ (about 1 cm)
C. 1″ (about 2.5 cm)
D. 1½″ (about 4 cm)

10 Which antibody contained in breast milk provides passive immunity for a neonate?

A. IgA
B. IgB
C. IgC
D. IgG

11 Which neonatal skin variation is characterized by a pink, papular rash with superimposed vesicles?

A. Mongolian spots
B. Erythema toxicum
C. Telangiectatic nevus
D. Harlequin sign

12 The umbilical cord consists of:

A. One artery and two veins
B. Two arteries and two veins
C. Two arteries and one vein
D. One artery and one vein

13 After birth, the umbilical stump usually dries and falls off within:

A. 1 to 5 days
B. 7 to 10 days
C. 2 to 3 weeks
D. 4 to 6 weeks

14 Which condition can result from an untreated maternal chlamydial infection?

A. Chronic conjunctivitis
B. Deafness
C. Vesicular lesions around the vagina
D. Hemolytic anemia

15 Cow's milk sensitivity in a neonate is manifested by:

A. Circumoral pallor
B. Excessive crying
C. Hypotonia
D. Tearing

16 Which of the following is an acceptable substitute for cow's milk in a milk-sensitive neonate?

A. Goat's milk
B. Evaporated milk
C. Soy formula
D. Powdered milk

17 Which term describes the vaguely outlined scalp edema that occurs in neonates?

A. Caput succedaneum
B. Cephalhematoma
C. Subdural hematoma
D. Petechiae

18 A neonate with sickle cell anemia is protected from initial morbidity because of:

A. Maternal antibodies
B. Persistent fetal circulation
C. Fetal hemoglobin
D. Maternal hemoglobin

19 Which precaution should the nurse take during transfusion of a neonate?

A. Increase the amount of saline as a primer in the tubing
B. Leave off the filter so that platelets do not become trapped
C. Use the largest gauge needle possible
D. Change the tubing and filter with every new unit of blood

20 A neonate who is receiving a double-volume exchange transfusion is at increased risk for all of the following complications *except:*

A. Acidemia
B. Hypokalemia
C. Hyperkalemia
D. Hypoglycemia

21 A neonate is at increased risk for all types of infection because of:

A. His decreased metabolic rate
B. The IgG maternal antibodies
C. The stress of birth
D. His immature and inexperienced immune system

SITUATION

Darlene, a 2-week-old premature neonate, is placed on total parenteral nutrition (TPN), consisting of an infusion of a hyperalimentation solution at 5 ml/hour and an intralipid solution at 0.1 ml/hour. A central venous line is also in place.

Questions 22 to 25 refer to this situation.

22 The nurse's primary concern in caring for Darlene is to:

A. Assess her vital signs every 30 minutes
B. Monitor her blood glucose level
C. Elevate the head of the bed 60 degrees
D. Provide a daily bath

23 The nurse is aware that TPN tubing should be changed every:

A. 8 hours
B. 24 hours
C. 48 hours
D. 72 hours

24 An elevation of which laboratory value signals a problem with Darlene's intralipid therapy?

A. Bilirubin
B. Sodium
C. Phosphate
D. Calcium

25 During Darlene's TPN infusion, the I.V. tubing becomes dislodged. The nurse's top priority is to:

A. Immediately notify the pediatrician
B. Turn off the infusion pump
C. Monitor Darlene's heart rate
D. Clamp the central venous line catheter tubing

SITUATION

Patrice, a 5-day-old small-for-gestational-age neonate weighing only 3¹/₄ lb (1,500 g) at birth, was born to a 35-year-old pre-eclamptic patient. Patrice's Apgar scores were 1 and 5 immediately after delivery, and her initial vital signs were: heart rate, 156 beats/minute; respiratory rate, 62 breaths/minute; temperature, 97.2° F (36.2° C); mean arterial pressure, 22 mm Hg; hematocrit, 72%; and blood glucose level, 130 mg/dl. Yesterday, Patrice was started on nasogastric feedings; today, she is lethargic, exhibits feeding intolerance, and has abdominal distention.

Questions 26 to 29 refer to this situation.

26 Which assessment finding indicates that Patrice is at risk for necrotizing enterocolitis (NEC)?

A. Hematocrit of 72%
B. Nasogastric feeding started on the fourth day after birth
C. Blood glucose level of 130 mg/dl
D. Heart rate of 156 beats/minute, respiratory rate of 62 breaths/minute, and temperature of 97.2° F (36.2° C)

27 Which sign (besides lethargy, feeding intolerance, and abdominal distention) suggests NEC?

A. Increased intracranial pressure
B. Bloody stools
C. Seizures
D. Hypertension

28 Which nursing action is most important for Patrice, who is at risk for NEC?

A. Positioning Patrice on her abdomen after each feeding
B. Suctioning Patrice every 4 hours
C. Recognizing and responding to changes in Patrice's color, tone, and general activity
D. Assessing Patrice's temperature rectally for early signs of infection

29 Which complication is most common in neonates with NEC?

A. Hydrocephalus
B. Pneumothorax
C. Cholecystitis
D. Intestinal perforation

SITUATION

Sean is delivered at 44 weeks' gestation by cesarean section because of fetal distress. At delivery, he has a thick, green-tinged coating, cyanosis, and signs of respiratory distress. The physician diagnoses meconium aspiration syndrome.

Questions 30 to 32 refer to this situation.

30 Which factor would predispose Sean to meconium aspiration syndrome?

A. Prematurity
B. Maternal sepsis
C. Postmaturity
D. Maternal diabetes

31 If the physician suspects that Sean has pneumothorax, the nurse should prepare to do all of the following *except:*

A. Assist with intubation
B. Assist with chest tube insertion
C. Encourage Sean to cry
D. Administer oxygen

32 Appropriate nursing measures for Sean include all of the following *except:*

A. Auscultating breath sounds frequently
B. Performing chest physiotherapy and suctioning
C. Monitoring oxygenation
D. Encouraging early oral feeding to maintain a normoglycemic state

SITUATION

Mrs. Johnson brings her 2-week-old son, Frank, to the pediatrician's office for a routine neonatal assessment. The history reveals that Frank was full-term and healthy, weighing 8 lb, 10 oz (3,912 g) at birth. He was delivered spontaneously and vaginally, with no maternal analgesia or anesthesia. Apgar scores were 9 and 10. After an uneventful hospital stay, Frank was discharged on the third postpartal day, weighing 8 lb, 4 oz (3,742 g). Mrs. Johnson, who is breast-feeding, reports that she is feeling tired and that Frank wants to feed "much too frequently." Physical assessment reveals an alert, hydrated 2-week-old neonate, weighing 8 lb, 10 oz (3,912 g).

Questions 33 to 35 refer to this situation.

33 When responding to Mrs. Johnson's complaint that Frank feeds too frequently, the nurse should:

A. Assess Mrs. Johnson's expectations regarding feeding frequency
B. Reassure Mrs. Johnson that a growing neonate needs to feed often
C. Tell Mrs. Johnson to space the feedings more appropriately
D. Review Mrs. Johnson's dietary history

34 When assessing Franks's weight, the nurse notes that:

A. The weight is acceptable
B. The weight indicates inadequate nutritional intake
C. The weight is the same as the birth weight, indicating a possible failure to thrive
D. The weight gain is excessive for the 2-week period

35 The stools of a healthy, exclusively breast-fed 2-week-old neonate are typically:

A. Greenish brown and semisolid, occurring once or twice a day
B. Easy to pass, but irritating to the neonate's sensitive skin
C. Yellowish, formed, and sweet-smelling
D. Yellowish and loose or watery, occurring at nearly every feeding

SITUATION

Mrs. Horn arrives at the well-child clinic with her son, Vincent, a healthy, exclusively breast-fed 4-week-old infant. Height and weight measurements place him in the 75th percentile for both parameters, where he has been since birth. Further nursing assessment reveals that Vincent exhibits age-appropriate growth and development.

Questions 36 to 38 refer to this situation.

36 Mrs. Horn asks the nurse to review Vincent's nutritional requirements. On which rationale should the nurse base her nutritional teaching?

A. Breast milk is a complete food that meets an infant's nutritional requirements
B. An infant should begin eating solid foods at age 4 weeks
C. An exclusively breast-fed 4-week-old infant requires additional fluid, so sterile water should be offered
D. All of the above

37 All of the following statements about milk extraction are true *except:*

A. Compression of the sinuses beneath the areola is one way the infant extracts milk
B. Suction applied to the nipple and areola is the only way to extract milk
C. The infant releases milk from the breast by stroking the areola with his tongue
D. Both manual expression and pumping are acceptable methods of extracting milk

38 Which statement about the storage of expressed breast milk is *true?*

A. Breast milk contains macrophages, which prevent bacterial growth when milk is stored and reheated
B. Breast milk is naturally homogenized
C. Breast milk should be stored in sterilized containers
D. Breast milk should be refrigerated, not frozen, and used within 48 hours

---

SITUATION

Min Yang, age 18 months, was diagnosed at birth with Down's syndrome. The youngest of four children, she is enrolled in an infant stimulation program sponsored by a local school district and attends sessions twice weekly with her mother, age 40. Min also sees an occupational therapist, a physical therapist, and a special education teacher.

Questions 39 to 44 refer to this situation.

39 Which nursing action is most appropriate after the parents of an infant with Down's syndrome first learn of the diagnosis?

A. Discuss the special programs available for children with Down's syndrome
B. Encourage an early decision about placing the infant in a special program
C. Recommend getting a second opinion
D. Emphasize the infant's positive normal characteristics

40 The respiratory tract infections typical of a patient with Down's syndrome usually are caused by:

A. Hypotonicity of chest muscles
B. Hypertonicity of chest muscles
C. Decreased oral secretions
D. Increased oral secretions

41 After extensive testing and evaluation, Min is classified as moderately retarded but trainable. Which statement best describes this classification?

A. Min may require life-long supervision, but she should be able to perform simple tasks, such as those in sheltered workshops
B. Min may be able to work in different situations and live an independent life, but she may need support during a crisis
C. Min may achieve some success in regular classroom settings, but she will need more time to achieve goals
D. None of the above

42 Which intervention is the nurse's priority when developing a plan of care for a child with Down's syndrome who requires constant bed rest?

A. Monitoring the child's height and weight
B. Emphasizing social interaction and play
C. Keeping the child's skin well lubricated
D. Assessing the child's ability to perform self-care

43 The nurse can promote Min's optimal development best by:

A. Assessing her development at 3-month intervals
B. Encouraging her to hold finger foods
C. Helping Mrs. Yang to set realistic goals for Min
D. Discussing home care options with Mrs. Yang

44 Which nursing intervention would best help Mrs. Yang with feeding solid foods?

A. Point out that tongue thrusting is a child's way of rejecting food
B. Instruct Mrs. Yang to place the food to the back and side of Min's mouth
C. Tell Mrs. Yang to puree the foods if Min resists them in solid form
D. Suggest force-feeding when necessary

Answer sheet

	A B C D		A B C D
1	○○○○	31	○○○○
2	○○○○	32	○○○○
3	○○○○	33	○○○○
4	○○○○	34	○○○○
5	○○○○	35	○○○○
6	○○○○	36	○○○○
7	○○○○	37	○○○○
8	○○○○	38	○○○○
9	○○○○	39	○○○○
10	○○○○	40	○○○○
11	○○○○	41	○○○○
12	○○○○	42	○○○○
13	○○○○	43	○○○○
14	○○○○	44	○○○○
15	○○○○		
16	○○○○		
17	○○○○		
18	○○○○		
19	○○○○		
20	○○○○		
21	○○○○		
22	○○○○		
23	○○○○		
24	○○○○		
25	○○○○		
26	○○○○		
27	○○○○		
28	○○○○		
29	○○○○		
30	○○○○		

Answers and rationales

1 Correct answer—**A**

Deoxyribonucleic acid (DNA) is a large nucleic acid molecule found primarily in chromosomes of the nucleus of the cells that carries the genetic code. A chromosome is a threadlike structure found in the nucleus of a cell that functions in the transmission of genetic information. Each cell normally contains 23 pairs of chromosomes—22 pairs of homologous chromosomes and 1 pair of sex chromosomes. A barr body is the inactivated X chromosome in the female pair of sex chromosomes that appears as a dark area on the edge of the cell. An autosome is any chromosome of the 22 pairs of homologous chromosomes in the nucleus of a cell that is not a sex chromosome.

2 Correct answer—**B**

A karyotype is a microphotographic representation of the chromosomes contained in the nucleus of a cell—normally 22 pairs of autosomes and 1 pair of sex chomosomes (XX or XY). The normal female karyotype is depicted as 46 chromosomes, consisting of 22 pairs of autosomes and 1 pair of sex (XX) chromosomes, which can be abbreviated as 46XX. The normal male karyotype is abbreviated as 46XY. Examples of abnormal karyotypes are 47XY (male with one extra chromosome) and 45XX (female with one missing chromosome).

3 Correct answer—**A**

For a homozygous recessive trait to occur, both parents, who are unaffected and heterozygous for the trait, must pass the defective gene or set of genes to the child. In each pregnancy, the child has a 25% chance of acquiring the trait, a 50% chance of being a carrier of the trait, and a 25% chance of being unaffected.

4 Correct answer—**D**

For autosomal dominant inheritance to occur, at least one parent must have the trait. Thus, affected persons always have an affected parent. Because a dominant gene always expresses itself, the parent can be heterozygous and still have the trait. Family histories are always positive for the trait, and both males and females are equally affected.

5 Correct answer—D

In X-linked recessive disorders, the daughters of an affected male are carriers of the trait. This situation occurs because males always inherit the Y chromosome of their fathers' sex chomosomes; females, the X chromosome, which contains the trait. The daughters then pass on the trait to their sons, who are affected with the disorder.

6 Correct answer—D

Phenylketonuria (PKU), an autosomal recessive disorder that causes mental retardation from increased levels of phenylalanine in the blood, can be controlled by a milk-free, low-protein diet when diagnosed early. Infants with PKU can be breast-fed (breast milk is normally low in phenylalanine) or fed a specially prepared formula. PKU is not controlled by insulin, pancreatin, or braces.

7 Correct answer—C

Trisomy 21, commonly known as Down's syndrome, is characterized by phenotypic features affecting the face (epicanthal folds, flat nasal bridge, and tongue protrusion), hands (simian creases), and muscle tone (hypotonia). The most common chromosomal disorder, trisomy 21 is associated with varying degrees of mental retardation, cardiac disease, and blood disorders. Trisomy 13, the severest of the trisomy disorders, is marked by a small head and eyes, seizures, and deafness. Trisomy 18, which affects nearly all organ systems, is characterized by a small head, low-set ears, and diminutive features. Trisomy 46 does not exist.

8 Correct answer—B

When studying hereditary patterns, researchers commonly refer to twins as being concordant or discordant (depending on the appearance of shared or unshared traits) and monozygous or dizygotic (depending on the fertilization process by which the twins originated). Concordant twins share the same genetically inherited trait, such as eye or hair color. Discordant twins do not share the same specific trait. Monozygous twins are identical, originating from a single fertilized ovum. Dizygotic, or fraternal, twins result from the fertilization of two ova by two sperm. Both monozygous and dizygotic twins can be concordant or discordant for specific traits.

9 Correct answer—C

To obtain an accurate rectal temperature in a neonate, the thermometer should be inserted 1″ (2.5 cm). Insertion of more than 1¼″ (3 cm) can cause trauma to the colon. Lubricating the tip of the thermometer helps to ease insertion.

10 Correct answer—A

Human breast milk contains immunoglobulin A (IgA), which provides passive immunity for the neonate against certain bacterial and viral infections, especially those affecting the respiratory and gastrointestinal systems. IgA also may play a role in the prevention of food allergies. IgG, which is transferred to the fetus via the placenta and stored in fetal tissues late in pregnancy, provides passive immunity against various infectious agents. IgB and IgC do not exist.

11 Correct answer—B

Erythema toxicum, marked by a pink, papular rash with superimposed vesicles, is a common neonatal skin variation. Mongolian spots are deep blue, irregular areas usually found in the sacral region. Telangiectatic nevus, commonly referred to as a stork bite, is a condition characterized by a flat, pink pigmented area on the neck or face. Harlequin sign, caused by vasomotor instability, results in reddening of the lower half of the body and blanching of the upper half when the neonate is placed on his side.

12 Correct answer—C

The umbilical cord consists of three blood vessels—two small arteries and one large vein. At birth, the cord appears bluish white and moist until it is clamped, at which time the vessels become apparent. Inspection of the cord at this time is important because cord anomalies may indicate birth defects. Usually, a dye solution or alcohol is applied to the cord to prevent infection and to aid in drying.

13 Correct answer—B

The umbilical stump usually dries and falls off within 7 to 10 days. The base of the cord, or stump, may take 2 weeks to heal completely. Keeping the stump area clean and dry helps to prevent infection, which is indicated by a malodorous, purulent discharge and erythema. Diapers should be positioned below the umbilicus to prevent irritation and to keep the area dry.

14 Correct answer—**A**

An untreated maternal chlamydial infection can cause chronic conjunctivitis, which the neonate acquires when coming in contact with the mother's infected cervix during the birth process. The conjunctivitis commonly resolves spontaneously, but scarring can occur. Chlamydial infection does not cause deafness, vesicular lesions, or hemolytic anemia.

15 Correct answer—**B**

Cow's milk sensitivity is commonly manifested by excessive crying, diarrhea, vomiting, colic, abdominal pain, and rhinitis. Eczema also may be related to this condition. Typically, such sensitivity becomes evident during the first 2 months or after the first ingestion of cow's milk by an infant who was exclusively breast-fed. By age 2, most children can tolerate cow's milk.

16 Correct answer—**C**

Commercially prepared soy formula is an acceptable substitute for an infant who is sensitive to cow's milk. Some infants also are sensitive to soy formula and require a hydrolyzed protein formula or an amino acid formula. Goat's milk is an unacceptable substitute because it can cross-react with cow's milk protein and is deficient in folic acid. Evaporated milk and powdered milk both contain a cow's milk base and therefore are unacceptable.

17 Correct answer—**A**

Caput succedaneum is a vaguely outlined scalp edema that crosses the suture line and typically clears within a few days after birth. Cephalhematoma is a swelling of the head that results from subcutaneous bleeding caused by pressure exerted on the soft tissues during delivery; it is characterized by sharply demarcated boundaries that do not cross the suture lines. Subdural hematoma is a collection of blood between the dura and the brain. Petechiae are minute, circumscribed hemorrhagic areas in the skin.

18 Correct answer—**C**

A neonate with sickle cell anemia is protected from initial morbidity because of high levels of fetal hemoglobin, which decline as he grows. By age 2, the child typically achieves adult hemoglobin configurations, and the sickling process increases. Maternal antibodies (IgG) transferred via the placenta provide passive immunity; however, they have no effect on the neonate's anemia. Maternal hemoglobin does not cross the placenta; therefore, it offers no protection against anemia. Persistent fetal circulation is associated with cardiac disease and results in hypoxia; it is unrelated to the sickling process.

19 Correct answer—D

During transfusion of a neonate or an infant, the nurse should change the tubing and filter with every new unit of blood to prevent contamination from untrapped cells, blood particles, or impurities that can lead to septicemia. Saline solution is used during transfusions to flush the tubing of any possible dextrose solution that can cause hemolysis of blood cells; however, the amount should not be increased for a neonate because of the neonate's inability to manage excess fluids within the circulatory system. All blood products must be filtered to prevent contamination; leaving off the filter to prevent platelets from becoming trapped would be inappropriate. Because of the size of the neonate's veins, the smallest gauge needle should be used.

20 Correct answer—B

A neonate receiving a double-volume exchange transfusion is at risk for a host of complications; however, hypokalemia is not among them. Potential complications include acidemia, hyperkalemia, hypoglycemia, perforation of the umbilical vein or artery, infection, intestinal perforation, hypothermia (especially if the blood is not prewarmed), and air embolism. Hyperkalemia, which is most likely to occur when donor blood is more than 4 days old, can lead to cardiac arrest; therefore, neonates and infants require electrocardiogram monitoring during the procedure. The nurse also should pay careful attention to the volume and speed of the transfusion.

21 Correct answer—D

Because of his relatively immature and inexperienced immune system, a neonate is at increased risk for all types of infection. IgG antibodies, acquired in utero, protect the neonate for 3 to 6 months from infections to which the mother is immune. The neonate's metabolic rate and birth experience do not affect his developing immune system, which protects him from infection. After birth, however, the developing immune system can be affected by various factors, such as exposure to bacterial flora.

22 Correct answer—B

The nurse's primary concern in this situation is to carefully monitor Darlene's blood glucose level. Because most hyperalimentation solutions used for total parenteral nutrition (TPN) contain a high glucose content, the neonate is at risk for hyperglycemia. A neonate receiving TPN usually does not require a vital signs assessment every 30 minutes nor does she need the head of the bed elevated 60 degrees. Providing a daily bath is not a primary nursing concern for this neonate.

23 Correct answer—B

TPN solutions containing protein are an excellent medium for the growth of microorganisms. To prevent infection, TPN tubing should be changed every 24 hours, and any remaining TPN solution should be discarded and a new solution bag used. Changing the solution at this time prevents too-frequent disruption of the I.V. system, further reducing the risk of infection and the introduction of an air embolism.

24 Correct answer—A

Because hyperbilirubinemia—excessive levels of bilirubin in the blood—is a contraindication to intralipid therapy, an elevated bilirubin value signals a problem with therapy. Thrombocytopenia also can occur during intralipid therapy, so a low platelet count is cause for concern. Hypernatremia (an excessive blood sodium level), hyperphosphatemia (an excessive blood phosphate level), and hypocalcemia (a decreased calcium level) usually occur during TPN therapy.

25 Correct answer—D

When a portion of tubing connected to a central venous line becomes dislodged, the nurse should immediately clamp the central venous line catheter tubing to prevent an air embolism. She then should notify the pediatrician and monitor the neonate's vital signs. Turning off the infusion pump is not the first priority in this case.

26 Correct answer—A

Necrotizing enterocolitis (NEC), an acute inflammatory bowel disorder, is characterized by necrosis of the small or large intestine caused by ischemic damage. This condition occurs because diminished perfusion to the intestinal wall causes the cells lining the intestine to stop secreting protective mucus, allowing for bacterial invasion. A polycythemic neonate has a reduced blood volume and typically shows signs of circulatory insufficiency. In this situation, Patrice has a hematocrit of 72%, indicating blood volume depletion, which can lead to ischemia of the bowel and subsequent development of NEC. Because early feeding (within the first 24 to 48 hours after birth) is associated with NEC, beginning nasogastric feedings on the fourth day is appropriate. The glucose level is unrelated to NEC. Although NEC can be caused by hypoxia, Patrice's vital signs do not suggest respiratory distress.

27 Correct answer—B

Frank or occult bloody stools usually signify a bowel injury and are characteristic of a neonate with NEC. Although the clinical signs typically are nonspecific and variable, most neonates with NEC exhibit progressive lethargy, feeding intolerance, abdominal distention, hypovolemia, bloody stools, and apnea. Increased intracranial pressure, seizures, and hypertension usually are not related to this disorder.

28 Correct answer—C

Patrice's prognosis can be greatly improved by careful observation for early signs and symptoms of NEC. Prompt medical intervention significantly reduces infant mortality and the need for surgery. Therefore, the nurse must be able to recognize and respond to minor, sometimes subtle, changes in color, tone, and general activity in a neonate at risk for NEC. Because a neonate with NEC exhibits abdominal distention, positioning Patrice on her abdomen would make assessment for this sign impossible. Because of the traumatic nature of suctioning, this procedure should be done only as needed and not on a rigid schedule. Although frequent monitoring of vital signs is necessary for detecting signs of sepsis, assessing Patrice's temperature rectally is contraindicated because of the increased risk of colon perforation.

29 Correct answer—D

The most common complication in neonates with NEC is intestinal perforation, which results from air buildup in the intestinal lining produced by invading gas-forming organisms. Hydrocephalus, pneumothorax, and cholecystitis are unrelated to NEC.

30 Correct answer—C

Sean is predisposed to meconium aspiration syndrome because of his postmaturity. A postmature neonate does not tolerate the stress of labor as well as a full-term neonate does and is more prone to asphyxiation. Uteroplacental functioning, already compromised because of postmaturity, also is adversely affected by the onset and duration of labor. Meconium aspiration syndrome is rare in premature neonates. Maternal sepsis does not affect uteroplacental function, except when the mother develops septic shock, which decreases blood flow to the uterus and placenta. Maternal diabetes is associated primarily with neonatal hypoglycemia and largeness for gestational age, not with meconium aspiration syndrome.

31 Correct answer—C

The immediate aims in treating a neonate with meconium aspiration syndrome are to clear the meconium from the neonate's airways and improve his oxygenation, gas exchange, and pulmonary function. Encouraging Sean to cry may force meconium particles into his airway, further compromising gas exchange and increasing the risk of pneumothorax. The nurse should be prepared to assist with intubation and chest tube insertion (to evacuate any accumulated air in the event of a pneumothorax) and to administer oxygen.

32 Correct answer—D

Although maintaining a normoglycemic state is imperative, oral feedings are contraindicated in a neonate who is intubated or exhibiting signs and symptoms of respiratory distress. Feeding is best accomplished through the use of I.V. infusions. Appropriate nursing interventions include obtaining a baseline respiratory reading, then frequently auscultating breath sounds for changes in respiratory status that might indicate a pneumothorax; performing chest physiotherapy to loosen particles of meconium in the neonate's airways, and suctioning; and monitoring for adequate oxygenation to ensure that the neonate does not suffer from further hypoxia, which can cause lung damage.

33 Correct answer—A

In this situation, the nurse should assess the mother's expectations regarding the frequency and duration of feedings. A healthy neonate who is breast-fed on demand usually feeds 10 to 12 times a day, or every 2 to 3 hours. If the neonate seems to require more frequent feedings, he may not be nursing long enough on each breast at each feeding. The nurse can instruct the mother to space the feedings more appropriately only after she reviews the neonate's usual schedule. Although reviewing the mother's diet is important to ensure that she is eating well-balanced meals that satisfy her increased nutritional needs during lactation, the neonate's feeding pattern is of greater concern in this case. Before reassuring the mother that a growing neonate needs to eat often, the nurse should first consider all the other factors related to the frequent feedings.

34 Correct answer—A

A healthy, full-term neonate usually experiences a 5% weight loss during the first 3 days after delivery when fed by a mother who is breast-feeding for the first time. A 10% weight loss may be acceptable if no other problems are evident; however, in such a situation, close monitoring is essential. Frank had a 6-oz (4%) weight loss at discharge, then regained his birth weight by age 2 weeks, indicating adequate intake and an acceptable weight.

35 Correct answer—D

The stools of an exclusively breast-fed neonate typically are yellowish and loose or watery, occurring at nearly every feeding. They usually are nonirritating to the skin and easy to pass. Because breast milk has a laxative effect during the first few weeks, the stools may appear seedy or have the consistency of cottage cheese. In some cases, peristalsis slows and the neonate does not defecate for several days to a week; the color and consistency of the stools, however, should remain the same.

36 Correct answer—A

Breast milk is a complete food that meets a young infant's nutritional requirements; it is the only food or fluid needed by a

healthy 1-month-old infant. A 1-month-old infant does not have
the oral motor skills necessary to consume solid food; also, the extrusion (tongue thrust) reflex is too strong to allow the neonate to
swallow solids. By age 6 months, the infant loses the extrusion reflex and acquires the oral motor capability needed to accept solids
from a spoon. Also, he can sit with support, his teeth have probably begun to erupt, and his digestive tract is mature enough to digest solid food. At this age, his nutritional requirements cannot be
met by breast milk alone and solid foods should be added to the
diet. Initially, the solid foods should contain iron in the form of
grains or iron-fortified cereals.

37 Correct answer—B

Applying suction to the nipple and areola is one way that an infant
extracts breast milk. He also can extract milk from the breast by
compressing the sinuses beneath the areola with his gums, applying suction to the breast, and stroking the areola with his tongue.
Both manual expression and pumping are acceptable methods of
extracting milk. Manual expression involves compressing the areola, which helps to release milk contained in the lactiferous
sinuses. Pumping involves suctioning, which sufficiently empties
foremilk from the breast.

38 Correct answer—C

Because the anti-infective properties of breast milk are decreased
by freezing and reheating, expressed breast milk should be col-
lected and stored in sterile containers. Plastic containers are preferred over glass because the leukocytes in freshly expressed
breast milk have been found to adhere to glass. Macrophages in
breast milk are characterized by ameboid movement and phago-
cytic and bactericidal properties. However, these cells are not via-
ble when the milk is heated to 145° F (63° C) or cooled to –9° F
(–23° C), and they lose their anti-infective effects with freezing
and reheating. Breast milk is not homogenized. The top layer of
expressed milk is cream and does not indicate curdling; mixing
the milk before feeding is unnecessary. Breast milk can be frozen
and stored up to 6 months.

39 Correct answer—D

Emphasizing the normal characteristics of an infant with Down's
syndrome helps to foster parental acceptance by giving the parents
something positive on which to focus. However, this does not

mean that abnormalities should be ignored. Because learning about the diagnosis of Down's syndrome can overwhelm the parents, the nurse should discuss the special programs available for children with Down's syndrome later, after the parents have had time to adjust to the news. The characteristic physical features of an infant with Down's syndrome are easy to detect and commonly serve as the basis for an initial diagnosis until genetic testing is completed. Recommending that the parents pursue a second opinion rather than seek confirmation of the diagnosis is inappropriate.

40 Correct answer—A

Down's syndrome is a genetically acquired disease that affects both sexes equally and usually results in mental retardation, congenital heart disease, and respiratory tract infections. A patient with Down's syndrome typically has weakened chest muscles; this hypotonicity prevents full lung expansion, which increases the risk of pooled secretions that can lead to respiratory infection. The amount of oral secretions is unrelated to respiratory tract infection (a patient with Down's syndrome typically has a normal amount of oral secretions).

41 Correct answer—A

A child classified as moderately retarded but trainable can perform simple tasks but may require supervision. Many children with Down's syndrome fit this classification; however, each child must be evaluated carefully. Because of the inability to perform complicated tasks or to participate in a complex and changing environment, independent living arrangements and regular classroom situations are unrealistic for these children.

42 Correct answer—C

Children with Down's syndrome typically have dry, rough skin that requires special attention to prevent breakdown, which can lead to infection, tissue loss, or deformity. Because constant bed rest increases the risk of skin breakdown, the nurse must keep the child's skin well lubricated. Although the other interventions are important, they are not the nurse's first priority.

43 Correct answer—C

The nurse can promote Min's optimal development best by helping Mrs. Yang to set realistic goals for her child. Ensuring that the goals are reasonable and attainable encourages the family members to work toward them together. Because of the physical deformities and potential for cognitive impairment associated with Down's syndrome, placing the child in an early intervention program is recommended to prevent health problems and maximize the child's developmental potential. Assessing the child at 3-month intervals instead of on an ongoing basis would not adequately meet Min's special needs. Holding finger foods is a normal developmental accomplishment for an 18-month-old; however, moderately retarded children experience significant delays in motor development. Thus, encouraging this activity may foster unrealistic expectations. Discussing home care options would be appropriate if the family rules out an early intervention program.

44 Correct answer—B

Placing food to the back and side of the child's mouth encourages swallowing. Tongue thrusting is a physiologic response to food that is placed incorrectly in the mouth and does not signify rejection of food. Swallowing solid foods is a learned behavior; feeding the child pureed food does not encourage this. Force-feeding can be frustrating for both the mother and child. It also can cause the child to gag and choke in an attempt to reject undesired food and can result in a higher-than-normal caloric intake that could lead to obesity.

CHAPTER 3

Assessment

Questions

1 A healthy neonate's respiratory rate ranges from:

A. 10 to 12 breaths/minute
B. 12 to 18 breaths/minute
C. 20 to 30 breaths/minute
D. 32 to 60 breaths/minute

2 Which pulse is best to assess in a neonate?

A. Apical
B. Brachial
C. Carotid
D. Pedal

3 A neonate demonstrates the tonic neck reflex by:

A. Extending the leg on the same side to which his head is turned
B. Flexing the leg on the same side to which his head is turned
C. Extending the leg on the opposite side to which his head is turned
D. Abducting the leg on the opposite side to which his head is turned

4 The best way for the nurse to examine a small child is by proceeding:

A. Cephalocaudally (head-to-toe)
B. Proximally to distally
C. From the most intrusive area to the least intrusive area
D. From the least intrusive area to the most intrusive area

5 Which measurement, besides height and weight, is commonly taken at each health assessment before age 2?

A. Head circumference
B. Chest circumference
C. Abdominal girth
D. All of the above

6 Which of the following best comforts a colicky infant?

A. Swaddling
B. Shaking
C. Giving an extra bottle
D. None of the above

7 During which activity can the nurse best assess infant-caregiver interaction?

 A. Sleeping
 B. Feeding
 C. Playing
 D. Rocking

8 Which cognitive milestone has a 10-month-old infant achieved when he searches for an object out of his visual range?

 A. Attentiveness
 B. Cognitive recall
 C. Symbolic learning
 D. Problem solving

9 When examining a neonate, the nurse measures and palpates the anterior fontanel. What information can be determined from this examination?

 A. Hydration status
 B. Neurologic status
 C. Cognitive status
 D. None of the above

10 Low-set ears in an infant may be associated with all of the following disorders *except:*

 A. Renal anomalies
 B. Otitis externa
 C. Down's syndrome
 D. Mental retardation

11 Which assessment finding might lead the nurse to suspect that an infant has been physically neglected?

 A. Dry skin
 B. Poor hygiene
 C. Weight gain
 D. Diarrhea

12 Which caregiver behavior would indicate a nursing diagnosis of *Knowledge deficit related to infant care?*

A. Ceasing to play with an infant when sensing his fatigue level
B. Limiting the self-feeding behaviors of an 11-month-old
C. Searching for additional ways to stimulate an infant
D. Establishing a demand feeding schedule in the early neonatal period

13 An enlarged scrotum in an infant younger than age 4 months indicates:

A. Hypospadias
B. Phimosis
C. Inguinal hernia
D. Hydrocele

14 Mrs. Evans, a first-time mother, asks the nurse if propping a bottle in her infant's mouth during a late-night feeding is acceptable. The nurse should respond that:

A. The infant may not receive adequate nutrition for growth with bottle propping; therefore, it is not recommended
B. The infant is capable of pushing away the bottle when satisfied; therefore, bottle propping is acceptable
C. The infant may develop otitis media from the bottle propping; therefore, it is not recommended
D. The infant receives enough stimulation and caregiver interaction with his other feedings; therefore, bottle propping during a late-night feeding is acceptable

15 The nurse discusses sibling rivalry with Mrs. Peters, whose second child recently was delivered. Which behavior might the mother expect her 3-year-old child to exhibit?

A. Advanced behavior for his age
B. Regressive behavior
C. Tantrums and sexual aggressiveness
D. Depression and apathy

16 All of the following neonates are at high risk for neonatal hypoglycemia *except:*

A. One who is small for gestational age
B. One whose mother is addicted to drugs
C. One who received an exchange transfusion 16 hours after birth
D. One who is undergoing phototherapy for hyperbilirubinemia

17 Children typically begin speaking in complete sentences between ages:

A. 1 and 1½
B. 2 and 2½
C. 2½ and 3
D. 4 and 5

18 A low-grade fever, barky cough, inspiratory stridor, and retractions in a child under age 3 may indicate:

A. Allergies
B. Asthma
C. Bronchitis
D. Croup

19 Which history finding is characteristic of a child who is enuretic after age 4?

A. Family history of enuresis
B. Calm temperament
C. Family's high socioeconomic status
D. Only-child status

20 When addressing the social and emotional needs of a school-age child, the nurse should focus on the child's:

A. Psychosexual development and knowledge of contraception
B. Self-esteem and feelings about his social responsibilities
C. Body image and feelings about his future adult responsibilities
D. None of the above

21 The school nurse examines a child with a sore throat and notes swollen anterior cervical nodes, a faint maculopapular rash, and a red pharynx. Which routine laboratory test would she expect the physician to order?

A. Throat culture
B. Nose culture
C. Complete blood count
D. Sputum culture

22 Varicella (chicken pox) lesions are characterized by:

A. An erythematous ring containing a white papule
B. An erythematous base with a fluid-filled vesicular top
C. A flat erythematous surface
D. A scaly erythematous surface

23 A child in which age-group is most susceptible to bone fractures?

A. Toddler
B. Preschooler
C. School-age child
D. Adolescent

24 When examining a school-age child's ear, the nurse must remember to pull the pinna:

A. Down and forward
B. Down and back
C. Up and back
D. Up and forward

25 The best way to assess an infant's thyroid gland is with the infant positioned:

A. Supine
B. Prone
C. Sitting
D. Standing

26 The neonatal hematocrit normally ranges from:

    A. 30% to 40%
    B. 31% to 43%
    C. 43% to 54%
    D. 45% to 65%

27 Hemoglobin levels in adolescent boys normally range from:

    A. 10 to 15 g/dl
    B. 11 to 16 g/dl
    C. 12 to 20 g/dl
    D. 14 to 18 g/dl

28 The bilirubin level of a normal 3- to 5-day-old neonate should not exceed:

    A. 2 mg/dl
    B. 6 mg/dl
    C. 8 mg/dl
    D. 12 mg/dl

29 When examining a school-age child or adolescent, the nurse should screen for which musculoskeletal deviation?

    A. Hip dysplasia
    B. Scoliosis
    C. Osteogenesis imperfecta
    D. All of the above

30 Robert, a 14-year-old black child, has irregular blue-pigmented areas on his buccal mucosa and gums. This condition may be described as a:

    A. Normal racial characteristic
    B. Physiologic response to lead ingestion
    C. Temporary hormonal manifestation common in adolescence
    D. Physiologic response to tetracycline exposure in childhood

31 Which examination tool is helpful in assessing the sexual maturity of an adolescent?

  A. Tanner Scale
  B. Denver Developmental Screening Test
  C. Dubowitz Scoring System
  D. Brazelton Scale

SITUATION

The public health nurse is checking on the progress of Mrs. Le Rue and Susan, her 2-week-old breast-fed daughter, who weighed 7 lb, 1 oz (3,203 g) at birth. After the nurse weighs Susan on a home infant scale at 8 lb (3,629 g), Mrs. Le Rue tells her that she is concerned that her daughter might not be getting enough breast milk. Mrs. Le Rue also mentions that she heard feeding cereal might help Susan to sleep better at night. The nurse learns through further questioning that Susan feeds every 3 to 4 hours for 20 to 25 minutes.

Questions 32 to 36 refer to this situation.

32 An appropriate response regarding the adequacy of breast milk would be:

  A. "Don't worry. Susan appears to be fine"
  B. "As long as Susan wets 6 to 8 diapers a day, she's receiving enough milk"
  C. "If your breasts are empty after the feedings, Susan is getting enough milk"
  D. "Weighing Susan after each feeding will determine whether she is getting enough milk"

33 At which age is cereal usually recommended?

  A. 6 weeks
  B. 8 weeks
  C. 4 months
  D. 6 months

34 While examining Susan's back, the nurse strokes the spinal area and observes for hip movement toward the stimulated side. This elicited reflex is called:

A. Dance
B. Crawling
C. Galant
D. Glabellar

35 The nurse notices small, yellow-white epithelial cysts near the midline of Susan's hard palate. These are known as:

A. Epstein's pearls
B. Uric acid crystals
C. Thrush spots
D. Milia

36 Mrs. Le Rue asks when the "soft spot" on top of Susan's head will disappear. The nurse replies that the anterior fontanel typically closes within:

A. 6 weeks
B. 12 weeks
C. 7 to 8 months
D. 9 to 18 months

SITUATION

Pamela Jeffries, age 4, is brought to the pediatric clinic by her mother for a mandatory physical examination for kindergarten placement. Mrs. Jeffries tells the nurse that although Pamela has been well since her last visit, she has a history of constipation, dental cavities, and anemia. The nurse checks Pamela's chart and notes that she also is a poor eater and is underweight.

Questions 37 to 43 refer to this situation.

37 When examining Pamela's abdomen, the nurse follows the proper assessment sequence of:

A. Palpation, inspection, auscultation, and percussion
B. Inspection, percussion, auscultation, and palpation
C. Inspection, auscultation, percussion, and palpation
D. Inspection, palpation, auscultation, and percussion

38 To correctly assess Pamela's bowel sounds, the nurse should auscultate:

A. Over the umbilicus
B. Over all four abdominal quadrants
C. At the epigastric area
D. Over the lower abdomen

39 The nurse would suspect appendicitis if Pamela has pain in which abdominal quadrant?

A. Right upper quadrant
B. Right lower quadrant
C. Left lower quadrant
D. Left upper quadrant

40 Which statement about liver palpation is *true?*

A. The liver can be felt in the right upper quadrant and should extend no more than 2″ (5 cm) below the right costal margin
B. The liver can be felt in the right lower quadrant and should extend no more than 1⅛″ (3 cm) below the right costal margin
C. The edge of the liver can be felt ⅜″ to ¾″ (1 to 2 cm) below the right costal margin in the right upper quadrant
D. The edge of the liver can be felt ⅜″ to ¾″ (1 to 2 cm) below the left costal margin in the left upper quadrant

41 Which is the most common palpable mass in a child's abdomen?

A. Wilms' tumor
B. Stool
C. Neuroblastoma
D. A cyst

42 Mrs. Jeffries tells the nurse that she has tried various methods to get Pamela to eat. Which approach might the nurse suggest?

A. Have Pamela eat alone
B. Offer Pamela a reward for eating
C. Serve Pamela portions smaller than those she would be expected to eat
D. Refuse to give Pamela any dessert if she does not eat

43 The pediatrician diagnoses Pamela as having an iron deficiency and prescribes ferrous sulfate. The nurse should instruct Mrs. Jeffries to:

A. Give the medication with meals
B. Watch for changes in Pamela's stool color
C. Increase Pamela's milk intake
D. All of the above

SITUATION

William, age 13, arrives at the clinic for a routine sports physical examination. His history reveals no serious illnesses or surgical procedures, and his immunizations are up to date. He is performing well in school and has no major physical complaints.

Questions 44 to 46 refer to this situation.

44 The nurse elicits additional information to complete her assessment of William. Which information would be *least* important in compiling data for such an examination?

A. William's endurance capabilities
B. Previous or current chronic illnesses
C. Neurologic or cardiovascular abnormalities
D. William's previous participation in group activities

45 Which area of the physical examination is *most* important in determining William's predisposition to injury?

A. Fundoscopic examination
B. Sexual maturity rating
C. Triceps skinfold measurement
D. Height and weight measurements

46 During the physical examination, the physician discovers that William has an arrhythmia and a slow heart rate and orders further testing. Which of the following would be necessary to determine conclusively William's ability to participate in sports?

A. Electrocardiogram
B. Exercise test
C. Chest X-ray
D. Complete blood count

Answer sheet

	A B C D		A B C D
1	○○○○	31	○○○○
2	○○○○	32	○○○○
3	○○○○	33	○○○○
4	○○○○	34	○○○○
5	○○○○	35	○○○○
6	○○○○	36	○○○○
7	○○○○	37	○○○○
8	○○○○	38	○○○○
9	○○○○	39	○○○○
10	○○○○	40	○○○○
11	○○○○	41	○○○○
12	○○○○	42	○○○○
13	○○○○	43	○○○○
14	○○○○	44	○○○○
15	○○○○	45	○○○○
16	○○○○	46	○○○○
17	○○○○		
18	○○○○		
19	○○○○		
20	○○○○		
21	○○○○		
22	○○○○		
23	○○○○		
24	○○○○		
25	○○○○		
26	○○○○		
27	○○○○		
28	○○○○		
29	○○○○		
30	○○○○		

Answers and rationales

1 Correct answer—**D**

A healthy neonate breathes between 32 and 60 times per minute. An obligate nose breather, he uses his abdominal muscles for respiration, which is frequently shallow and irregular. To determine an accurate rate, the nurse should count the respiratory rate for 1 minute during assessment.

2 Correct answer—**A**

Auscultating the apical area is the most accurate way to determine the rate and quality (rhythm, strength, and sound) of a neonate's pulse. The apical pulse, which should be assessed for 1 minute when the neonate is quiet, normally ranges from 110 to 160 beats/minute. Auscultating any of the other sites would yield imprecise results; a neonate has small arteries and a rapid pulse rate, which makes palpation of the pulse difficult.

3 Correct answer—**A**

The tonic neck reflex is demonstrated by extension of the leg on the same side to which the neonate's head is turned and by flexion of the contralateral arm and leg (asymmetrical positioning). This reflex typically disappears by age 3 or 4 months, when symmetrical positioning (movement of the limbs in unison) occurs.

4 Correct answer—**D**

When examining a small child, the nurse should proceed from the least intrusive area to the most intrusive area. Least intrusive areas are those that are readily accessible and least likely to provoke an anxious response in the child (for example, auscultating breath sounds while the child is held in the mother's lap). Intrusive areas are those that cause anxiety or discomfort (for example, examining the ears with an otoscope or palpating painful areas); these procedures should be conducted at the end of the examination.

5 Correct answer—**A**

The head circumference, along with height and weight, should be measured at each assessment before age 2. Head circumference usually measures between 12½" and 15" (32 and 38 cm) at birth, the head typically being one to two times larger than the chest. Delayed growth or failure to grow in height, weight, or head circumference is an early indication of a serious condition that requires immediate medical attention. Chest circumference and abdominal girth are not routinely assessed in a healthy child because these measurements do not provide additional data about the child's growth. However, in a child with a disorder, these measurements may provide important information about the child's condition (for example, measuring abdominal girth to assess ascites in a child with hepatic dysfunction).

6 Correct answer—**A**

A colicky infant responds best to swaddling, rocking, or sucking on a pacifier. Colic, a result of paroxysmal abdominal cramping or pain, causes the infant to cry loudly and draw his legs upward. Shaking the infant will not relieve the pain and may even cause trauma (shaken baby syndrome). Cow's milk sensitivity should be suspected in a formula-fed colicky infant; therefore, giving an extra bottle may exacerbate the problem.

7 Correct answer—**B**

Infant-caregiver interaction is best assessed during feeding. The way in which the caregiver holds the infant and looks at his face provides clues about her anxiety level and overall feelings for the child. Likewise, the infant's posture and responses to the caregiver provide clues about his comfort level and feelings. During feeding, the caregiver holds the infant close, usually within 12" to 15" of eye level. This distance seems most comfortable for the caregiver and provides the infant with optimal visual stimulation. Sleep periods do not provide an opportunity for infant-caregiver interaction. Although playing and rocking provide clues about developing infant-caregiver interaction, they are not the primary method of assessing such an exchange.

8 Correct answer—**C**

A 10-month-old infant demonstrates symbolic learning, the ability to envision an object after it is hidden or removed from view, when he searches for something out of his visual range. This activity also demonstrates that object permanence has been established. Attentiveness (the ability to respond to a stimulus) and cognitive recall (memory) usually are well established during the neonatal period. Problem solving is a concept too sophisticated for a 10-month-old infant.

9 Correct answer—**A**

Measuring and palpating the anterior fontanel, which normally is open in a neonate, can determine the neonate's hydration status; a depressed fontanel may indicate dehydration. Slight pulsations at the fontanel are common, but marked pulsations may be a sign of increased intracranial pressure. Cognitive and neurologic status are best assessed by checking the neonate's reflexes, sucking and swallowing coordination, vital signs, and gaze.

10 Correct answer—**B**

The top of the ear usually is located along an imaginary line drawn from the inner canthus of the eye to the outer canthus and extending to the ear. When the ears are located below this line, they are described as low-set. Otitis externa is an infection of the external auditory canal and is not related to ear placement. Renal anomalies, Down's syndrome, and mental retardation may be characterized by low-set ears.

11 Correct answer—**B**

Poor hygiene, skin infections (especially in the diaper area), and a flat occiput with a "bald spot" are probable signs of physical neglect. Weight loss or no weight gain also may be a sign of neglect. Dry skin and diarrhea do not necessarily indicate that the child has not been cared for. In most states, nurses must report all cases of suspected or actual abuse or neglect to a child welfare agency for further investigation.

12 Correct answer—**B**

A caregiver should encourage independent feeding behaviors in older infants. By age 9 months, an infant has sufficient neuromuscular development to allow him to eat finger foods, reach for foods, and drink from a cup. Therefore, limiting an 11-month-old infant's self-feeding indicates a *Knowledge deficit related to infant care*. The other options demonstrate appropriate infant care and parenting skills.

13 Correct answer—**D**

In an infant younger than age 4 months, an enlarged scrotum typically is caused by a hydrocele, an accumulation of fluid in the tunica vaginalis testis or along the spermatic cord; this condition resolves spontaneously within the first 3 months. After age 4 months, a palpable mass in the scrotum may be caused by an indirect inguinal hernia (protrusion of the intestines into the scrotal sac through a defect in the lumen of the processus vaginalis), which requires surgery. Hypospadias is a congenital defect in which the opening to the urinary meatus is on the underside of the penis. Phimosis is a condition in which the tightness of the foreskin prevents its retraction over the glans.

14 Correct answer—C

Bottle propping is not recommended because it places the infant at risk for otitis media, which results from a bacterial infection of the eustachian tube caused by the pooling of milk in the pharynx. An infant receives the same nutrition regardless of how the bottle is positioned. If the infant is not capable of pushing a propped bottle away, he could be at risk for aspiration. Bottle propping does not permit the close human contact, stimulation, and infant-caregiver interaction that normally occurs when an infant is held; from a psychosocial viewpoint, bottle-propping is inadvisable.

15 Correct answer—B

An older brother or sister experiencing sibling rivalry may display regressive, not advanced, behavior (baby talk, thumb sucking, or bed wetting); general aggressive behavior toward the new infant (taking toys, pulling hair, or hitting); misbehavior to attract parental attention (breaking toys, refusing to cooperate, or expressing negativism); and demanding or clingy behavior. Sibling rivalry usually is characterized by manifestations of overt jealousy and not by depression, apathy, or sexual aggressiveness, which indicate emotional or psychological problems. Tantrums (screaming, kicking, or lying on the floor in response to restrictions or unmet wishes) are a normal means of exerting independence during the toddler years.

16 Correct answer—D

A neonate undergoing phototherapy for hyperbilirubinemia is not at risk for neonatal hypoglycemia. Phototherapy reduces serum levels of unconjugated bilirubin and has no effect on glucogenesis. A small-for-gestational-age neonate has a diminished ability to produce glucose and therefore is at increased risk for hypoglycemia. A neonate whose mother is addicted to drugs may experience perinatal stress (drug withdrawal), which increases his metabolic needs relative to his glycogen stores, placing him at risk for hypoglycemia. A neonate who received an exchange transfusion 16 hours after birth may become hypoglycemic because stored red blood cells contain excessive glucose, which stimulates the insulin production that can lead to hypoglycemia.

17 Correct answer—C

Between ages 2½ and 3, a child typically undergoes accelerated development of vocabulary skills, verbal comprehension, and cognitive skills, resulting in an ability to link words to form complete sentences. A child uses about 400 words by age 2 and about 900 words by age 3.

18 Correct answer—D

In children under age 3, croup—an acute inflammatory condition of the upper and lower respiratory tracts that usually occurs in late fall and early winter—typically manifests as a low-grade fever, barky cough, inspiratory stridor, and retractions. Hoarseness and irritability also are common. Treatment includes increased fluids, humidification, and emotional support. Allergies, which are hypersensitive reactions to intrinsically harmless antigens (such as dust or pollen), are highly individualized and cause various symptoms. Asthma, a respiratory condition usually caused in a young child by inhalation of an allergen, is characterized by wheezing and dyspnea. Bronchitis can occur before age 4. Commonly associated with upper and lower respiratory tract infections, bronchitis is characterized by a dry, hacking, nonproductive cough that worsens at night and becomes productive after 2 to 3 days. Others symptoms include rhonchi and a slight fever.

19 Correct answer—A

A child who is enuretic after age 4 usually has a family history of enuresis (bed wetting); typically, one of the parents was enuretic as a child. Enuresis is most common in children from lower socioeconomic families, in boys who are members of large families, and in children who are tense or high-strung. Enuresis that resumes after a period of dryness may result from a urologic condition; evaluation is required in such cases.

20 Correct answer—B

The social and emotional needs of a school-age child (ages 6 to 12) typically center on self-esteem and social responsibility. During this developmental stage, caregivers should be sensitive to the child's need to bolster his self-esteem, develop a sense of responsibility to society, and become involved in community activities. A 6- to 12-year-old child is not typically concerned with psychosexual development or knowledge of contraception; these issues are too complex and future-oriented. Although a school-age child is interested in his physical appearance and may begin exploring his body parts out of curosity, the concept of body image does not become meaningful until adolescence, when the child begins to consider his future adult responsibilities.

21 Correct answer—A

A sore throat, swollen anterior cervical nodes, a faint maculopapular rash, and a red pharynx are associated with scarlet fever, a serious condition that sometimes manifests after a streptococcal infection. In light of such manifestations, the nurse would expect the physician to order a throat culture to check for group A beta-hemolytic streptococci. A positive culture accompanying the rash confirms the diagnosis. A nose culture, complete blood count, and sputum culture are unnecessary.

22 Correct answer—B

Varicella lesions have an erythematous base with a fluid-filled vesicular top; they usually are concentrated on the trunk and diminish in number distally. Patients are considered contagious 2 days before to 6 days after the rash appears; however, the lesions may take up to 2 weeks to clear completely.

23 Correct answer—C

A child is most susceptible to bone fractures during his school-age years, especially between ages 6 and 10, when his bones are growing faster than his muscles and ligaments. A child typically remains awkward and clumsy, and therefore susceptible to falls and other injuries, until his large and small muscle groups become more refined and enable him to develop greater strength and better coordination.

24 Correct answer—C

Anatomic ear variations are age-related. In children ages 3 and older, the eustachian tube and tympanic membrane are sloped vertically and the canal curves down and forward. The correct method for visualizing the tympanic membrane is to pull the pinna up and back. In infants and children under age 3, the eustachian tube and tympanic membrane slant horizontally and the external auditory canal curves upward. Thus the pinna should be pulled down and back to straighten the canal for viewing the tympanic membrane.

25 Correct answer—A

The best way to assess an infant's thyroid gland is to hyperextend the infant's neck slightly while he is in a supine position on the caregiver's lap. Using this approach, the caregiver can assist by stabilizing the infant's head. Hyperextending the neck helps the nurse to elongate the surface area of the infant's characteristically short neck to facilitate thyroid palpation. During thyroid assessment, the nurse also should examine the child's facial characteristics to determine whether his features correspond to his age; for example, infantile features in an older child may indicate cretinism (juvenile hypothyroidism, a chronic condition caused by insufficient thyroid secretion and marked by delayed eruption of teeth, excess weight, and difficulty performing cognitive tasks.) The nurse should examine an older child while he is seated, in the same manner as for an adult.

26 Correct answer—D

The neonatal hematocrit normally ranges from 45% to 65%, provided the umbilical cord is clamped immediately after delivery and is not stripped; stripping (applying manual pressure to the cord to force any remaining blood into the neonate) can result in hypervolemia.

27 Correct answer—D

Hemoglobin levels in adolescent boys normally range from 14 to 18 g/dl. The range for adolescent girls is lower, usually 12 to 16 g/dl.

28 Correct answer—D

The bilirubin level of a normal 3- to 5-day-old neonate should not exceed 12 mg/dl (normal levels are 2 to 12 mg/dl). A level higher than 12 mg/dl indicates physiologic jaundice; treatment typically includes phototherapy and the administration of oral or I.V. fluids to help excrete bilirubin through the urine and feces. Close monitoring of hydration status is necessary because exposure to the phototherapy lights can cause significant water loss.

29 Correct anwer—B

Screening for scoliosis, a lateral curvature of the spine, should be part of the physical examination in school-age children and adolescents. Scoliosis is a common problem in children, especially girls. Hip dysplasia (congenital hip dislocation) and osteogenesis imperfecta (a genetic disorder characterized by brittle bones that are highly susceptible to fracture) are congenital abnormalities of the musculoskeletal system that are evident at birth. Both disorders are treated during infancy.

30 Correct answer—A

Irregular, blue-pigmented areas on the buccal mucosa and gums are a normal racial characteristic of a 14-year-old black child. Many variations in skin color, hair pattern, buccal mucosa, and gum pigmentation can be attributed to race—for example, black children frequently have a bluish hue to the gums and buccal mucosa; black and Asian infants commonly have dark-blue pigmented areas (mongolian spots) in the sacral region that typically fade with age. The pigmentation described in this situation cannot be attributed to any of the other options listed.

31 Correct answer—A

The Tanner Scale, which stages adolescent sexual maturation, enables the nurse to determine the child's level of maturity by evaluating breast size, penis and scrotal size, and axillary and genital hair distribution. The Denver Developmental Screening Test, the Dubowitz Scoring System, and the Brazelton Scale are tools designed for assessing neonates and young children.

32 Correct answer—B

One of the most reliable indicators of whether a neonate is receiving an adequate amount of breast milk is the neonate's wetting 6
to 8 diapers a day. During the first few weeks of breast-feeding, a
mother's body begins to establish a milk supply that matches her
neonate's feeding habits; at this time, the neonate may be getting
enough milk even though the mother's breasts are not completely
empty. Considering the number of feedings and Mrs. Le Rue's
other neonatal and self-care responsibilities, weighing Susan after
each feeding would be unrealistic. Offering reassurance without
explaining how to determine whether Susan is getting enough
milk would not provide Mrs. Le Rue with the necessary information to ensure proper nutrition.

33 Correct answer—D

Cereal is not recommended before age 6 months because early introduction of solids to the infant's immature gastrointestinal system may lead to the development of food allergies. Also, the extrusion (tongue thrust) reflex, which normally pushes food out of the
mouth, remains strong before age 6 months. When solid foods finally are introduced, the usual sequence is rice cereal, which is
high in iron and easy to digest, followed by strained fruits and vegetables. Barley cereal, oatmeal, and meats can be added to the diet
later.

34 Correct answer—C

Movement of the hip toward the stimulated side is called trunk in-
curvation, or the galant reflex. This reflex normally disappears by
age 4 weeks. The dance, or step, reflex is elicited by holding the
neonate over a table or the floor and allowing her feet to touch the
hard surface; normally, the neonate responds by simulating a walking or dancing motion. The crawling reflex is evoked by placing
the neonate on her abdomen, which normally causes her extremities to move in a crawling motion. The glabellar reflex is elicited
when the bridge of the neonate's nose is briskly tapped, causing
her eyes to close.

35 Correct answer—A

Epstein's pearls, small epithelial cysts located on the neonate's
hard palate, are insignificant and typically disappear after a few

weeks. Uric-acid crystals, orange precipitates found on a neonate's diaper after urination, are common and of no clinical significance. Thrush, or oral candidiasis, appears as white patchy spots in a neonate's mouth; this fungal infection is contracted during a vaginal delivery when the mother is infected with vaginal candidiasis. Milia are small white papules commonly found on a neonate's chin, nose, and cheeks; these papules are distended sebaceous glands that usually disappear in a few weeks.

36 Correct answer—D

The anterior fontanel, located at the junction of the coronal, sagittal, and frontal sutures, normally closes between 9 and 18 months. At birth, this fontanel is diamond-shaped and usually measures 1″ to 2″ (2.5 to 5 cm). The posterior fontanel, which is triangular, is located at the sagittal and lambdoidal junction and normally closes by age 2 months. This fontanel, which may not be readily palpable at birth, usually measures 1/4″ to 3/8″ (0.5 to 1 cm).

37 Correct answer—C

When performing an abdominal examination, the nurse should follow the proper sequence of inspection, auscultation, percussion, and palpation. Palpating or percussing before auscultating may alter the loudness, pitch, or location of bowel sounds.

38 Correct answer—B

The nurse should auscultate over all four abdominal quadrants (right upper, right lower, left upper, and left lower) when assessing a child's bowel sounds. To assess for bowel sounds, which normally are characterized by gurgles and clicks, the nurse should press the diaphragm of the stethescope firmly against the child's abdomen and listen, noting the presence, quality, and frequency of sounds. Absent or decreased frequency of bowel sounds may indicate an obstructive disorder; increased frequency of bowel sounds usually indicates hyperperistalsis. The nurse can use the bell of the stethoscope to assess for sounds associated with the abdominal vasculature; the pulsation of the aorta usually can be auscultated over the epigastric region. Detection of abnormal sounds, such as murmurs, hums, and rubs, in this region should be reported to the physician.

39 Correct answer—B

The nurse should suspect appendicitis if Pamela has pain in the right lower quadrant of the abdomen. Other indications of appendicitis are pain in the periumbilical area, nausea and vomiting, constipation or diarrhea, and a mild fever.

40 Correct answer—C

The edge of the liver can be felt ⅜″ to ¾″ (1 to 2 cm) below the right costal margin in the right upper quadrant. Palpation of the liver beyond 1⅛″ (3 cm) indicates that the organ is enlarged. The spleen can be felt ⅜″ to ¾″ (1 to 2 cm) below the left costal margin in the left upper quadrant.

41 Correct answer—B

Stool, the most common palpable mass in a child's abdomen, usually is concentrated in the left lower quadrant, particularly in the descending colon. Occasionally, soft, gas-filled masses may be palpable in the right lower quadrant, in the cecum. When a child is constipated, stool and gas fill the left side of the colon to the ileocecal valve, causing pain in the right lower quadrant. Although Wilms' tumor (a malignant tumor of the kidney), neuroblastoma (a malignant tumor that commonly arises from the adrenal medulla), and cysts can manifest as abdominal masses, they are not the most common causes of a palpable mass in the lower left abdominal quadrant.

42 Correct answer—C

One effective measure to increase Pamela's food intake is to serve smaller portions, which prevent her from being overwhelmed by and unable to consume what is placed in front of her. Providing small portions is equivalent to setting small goals, which are more attainable to a child. Other measures to encourage eating include allowing Pamela to help with meal preparation, maintaining a calm environment, avoiding snacks, and providing rest periods before meals. Preparing simple menus, serving mildly seasoned food, and cutting food into small pieces also can help. Coaxing, bribing, threatening, or punishing a child should be avoided because she will learn to equate food with good or bad behavior, which could lead to emotional problems (such as anorexia nervosa) or obesity.

43 Correct answer—B

Because iron turns stools black, the nurse should instruct Mrs. Jeffries to watch for changes in Pamela's stool color to ensure that the supplements have been sufficiently absorbed. Iron supplements should be given between meals for better absorption; giving them shortly after meals helps to reduce gastric irritation. Increasing Pamela's milk intake may interfere with iron absorption; however, giving the medication with juices is recommended because vitamin C enhances iron absorption.

44 Correct answer—D

In this situation, the elicited information should be sports-oriented and include data necessary to determine William's suitability for participation in an athletic program. Information about previous participation in group activities, although somewhat helpful, is not necessary for this type of evaluation. Appropriate information should include William's endurance capabilities, any previous or current chronic illnesses, neurologic or cardiovascular abnormalities, history of fainting or loss of consciousness, previous injuries, medication use, immunization history, and family history of illness.

45 Correct answer—B

Rating an adolescent's degree of sexual maturation is crucial to determining his safe participation in sports. Based on Tanner's five stages of pubertal development, which encompass sexual and physical development, a child can be classified according to his risk for physical injury. For example, boys in Tanner's stages II and III (ages 11 to 14) typically vary in body size and strength; however, they still are considered skeletally immature and prone to epiphyseal injuries. For this reason, collision sports (such as football, rugby, and hockey) and contact sports (such as lacrosse, baseball, soccer, basketball, and wrestling) may be inappropriate for most boys at this developmental level; noncontact sports (such as swimming, certain track events, and racket sports) would be more appropriate. A fundoscopic examination reveals the status of the inner eye only; it does not assess visual acuity, which would be beneficial in this situation. Triceps skinfold measurements and height and weight measurements are important evaluative tools, but these findings alone cannot predict a child's injury potential.

46 Correct answer—**B**

Premature atrial or ventricular beats are the most common cause of adolescent arrhythmias. In teenagers, these findings commonly are associated with a slow heart rate. To better evaluate the effect of exercise on a child with such an arrhythmia, the physician should order an exercise test, which can be performed in the physician's office. This test simulates an exercise situation, which allows evaluation of the body's cardiovascular and respiratory responses to exercise. The child may be asked to climb stairs or run in place to the count of 50 steps. If the arrhythmia decreases as the heart rate exceeds 140 beats/minute, the child can safely participate in sports; if the arrhythmia persists, the child may require further evaluation by a cardiologist. During the test, the child's respiratory rate and effort can be assessed for signs of dyspnea upon exertion. An electrocardiogram does not reveal respiratory tolerance for exercise and, therefore, is limited in determining the child's ability to participate in sports. Neither a chest X-ray nor a complete blood count can assess cardiac and respiratory functioning.

CHAPTER 4

Sexual Concerns

Questions

1 A child's gender identity typically is established between ages:

A. 1 and 2
B. 2 and 4
C. 4½ and 8
D. 8 and 10

2 Follicle-stimulating hormone in males promotes:

A. Spermatozoa production
B. Spermatozoa maturation
C. Semen production
D. Testosterone release

3 In pubescent boys, pubic hair growth begins at the base of the:

A. Scrotum
B. Penis
C. Scrotum and penis
D. Inguinal lymph glands

4 Cryptorchidism is characterized by:

A. Testicular torsion
B. Testicular tumors
C. Testicular inflammation
D. Undescended testes

SITUATION

Rory, age 14, discusses birth control with the nurse during a routine visit to the adolescent clinic. She has been sexually active with the same boyfriend for about 6 months. Her last menstrual period was 2 weeks ago. The physician prescribes an oral contraceptive containing estrogen and progestin (Ortho-Novum).

Questions 5 to 9 refer to this situation.

5 Estrogen prevents pregnancy by:

A. Enhancing the midcycle peak of luteinizing hormone
B. Increasing the amount of progesterone secreted before ovulation
C. Inhibiting the release of follicle-stimulating hormone
D. Increasing the amount of progesterone released after ovulation

6 When advising Rory about birth control, the nurse should:

A. Stress the importance of abstinence
B. Discuss the health risks associated with each birth control method
C. Discuss the importance of sharing birth control information with her parents
D. Advise her that the most reliable method is an intrauterine device

7 Rory expresses concern about the risk of becoming pregnant while taking a combination-type oral contraceptive. The nurse tells her that, when taken properly, such a contraceptive is effective:

A. 88% of the time
B. 89% of the time
C. 91% of the time
D. 99% of the time

8 Which assessment finding is a contraindication for using a combination-type oral contraceptive?

A. Hypertension
B. Chronic otitis media
C. Idiopathic scoliosis
D. Hansen's disease

9 The nurse explains to Rory that the usual procedure for a missed dose of an oral contraceptive is to:

A. Discontinue taking the contraceptive for the remainder of the month
B. Take the missed dose as soon as she remembers, and take the next dose at the regularly scheduled time
C. Take the missed dose along with the next dose at the next regularly scheduled time
D. Take an extra dose to ensure protection

SITUATION

Amy Giordano, age 12, arrives at the emergency department with her mother, complaining of pain in her genital area. During the physical examination, Amy states that her stepfather has been forcing her to have sex with him for the past several months. The physician diagnoses genital herpes.

Questions 10 to 12 refer to this situation.

10 Which factor is commonly associated with incest?

A. Race
B. Social status
C. Ethnic background
D. Marital discord

11 The nurse should suspect genital herpes in a girl with:

A. Vesicular lesions in the genital area
B. Macular lesions in the genital area
C. Vaginal discharge resembling cottage cheese
D. Vaginal bleeding

12 Which statement about genital herpes is true?

A. It can be effectively treated with I.V. penicillin
B. It can be effectively treated with cryotherapy
C. It is curable and self-limiting
D. It is incurable, but medications can alleviate its discomfort

---

SITUATION

Sharon, age 15, reports to the school health office with complaints of lower abdominal pain and burning on urination.

Questions 13 to 18 refer to this situation.

---

13 Sharon tells the nurse that she recently noticed a vaginal discharge. Which characteristic about the discharge is most important for the nurse to record?

A. Color
B. Consistency
C. Odor
D. All of the above

---

14 The nurse elicits information about Sharon's sexual history. Which factor is essential to such a history?

A. Medication use
B. Physical development
C. Psychosocial development
D. Family history

---

15 During the interview, Sharon states that she has been sexually active with her boyfriend during the past 2 weeks. Based on this information, the nurse should ask:

A. "How long have you been sexually active without using a contraceptive?"
B. "What type of contraceptive are you using?"
C. "Does your boyfriend have similar symptoms?"
D. "Do your parents know about the relationship?"

---

16 Sharon tells the nurse that neither she nor her boyfriend uses any form of contraception. Which reason for not using a contraceptive is most commonly offered by adolescents?

A. They do not want their parents to know that they are sexually active
B. They deny that pregnancy is possible
C. They do not know about reproductive physiology
D. They prefer that sex be spontaneous

17 *Chlamydia,* a bacterial infection with both bacterial and viral characteristics, can be treated effectively with:

A. Penicillin
B. Ceftriaxone
C. Tetracycline
D. Amoxicillin

18 All of the following conditions can result from a sexually transmitted disease *except:*

A. Urinary tract infection
B. Pneumonia
C. Ectopic pregnancy
D. Sepsis

SITUATION

Laura Abrams, age 15, arrives with her mother at the hospital's outpatient clinic complaining of nausea, vomiting, and abdominal discomfort. Mrs. Abrams tells the nurse that Laura might have an influenza virus because another family member with similar complaints was diagnosed with the flu. A preliminary abdominal examination reveals nothing abnormal except for minimal lower quadrant tenderness. When questioned about her menstrual history, Laura responds that her periods are usually irregular.

Questions 19 to 21 refer to this situation.

19 Which information would be most important in further assessing Laura's symptoms?

A. The date of her last menstrual period
B. Her history of sexual activity
C. Her dietary history
D. The time of day vomiting usually occurs

20 Which interview technique would elicit the most accurate patient history in this situation?

A. Questioning Laura's mother
B. Questioning Laura and her mother simultaneously
C. Asking Laura's mother to wait outside the room while Laura is examined
D. Having Laura fill out a questionnaire

21 Based on the history and physical findings, the physician orders a pregnancy test, which is positive. Which reaction is typical of a 15-year-old who has just learned she is pregnant?

   A. Calm acceptance
   B. Readiness to make long-range plans
   C. Excitement and anticipation
   D. Denial or disbelief

SITUATION

June Scully, age 13, tells the clinic nurse that she has felt constantly fatigued and mildly nauseated over the past month and attributes these symptoms to mononucleosis. When asked about her menstrual history, she states that she has not had a period in about 2 months. A physical examination reveals that she is pregnant.

Questions 22 to 26 refer to this situation.

---

22 The initial nursing action should focus on:

   A. Helping June to plan a nutritious diet
   B. Discussing the growth and development of the fetus
   C. Setting up a schedule of clinic visits
   D. Assessing June's feelings about the pregnancy

23 According to Piaget, June may have difficulty making long-range plans about the birth of her child because she is still functioning at which level of cognitive development?

   A. Sensorimotor stage
   B. Preoperational stage
   C. Concrete operational stage
   D. Formal operational stage

24 In planning an optimum diet for June, the nurse should take into account which statement?

A. The high-carbohydrate diet favored by many teenagers can enhance the growth and development of the fetus
B. The adolescent's normal growth needs must be evaluated before planning any prenatal diet
C. By adolescence, most girls have adopted healthy eating habits
D. Most adolescents who become pregnant are already overweight and should be placed on restrictive diets

25 The demands of pregnancy require an additional caloric intake of:

A. 200 calories/day
B. 300 calories/day
C. 400 calories/day
D. 500 calories/day

26 Which strategy is *least* effective in teaching parenting skills to adolescents?

A. One-on-one demonstration and return demonstration, using a live infant as a model
B. Initiating an adolescent-parent support group with first- and second-time mothers
C. Using audiovisual aids that discuss skills and feelings
D. Providing age-appropriate reading materials

Answer sheet

A B C D
1 ○○○○
2 ○○○○
3 ○○○○
4 ○○○○
5 ○○○○
6 ○○○○
7 ○○○○
8 ○○○○
9 ○○○○
10 ○○○○
11 ○○○○
12 ○○○○
13 ○○○○
14 ○○○○
15 ○○○○
16 ○○○○
17 ○○○○
18 ○○○○
19 ○○○○
20 ○○○○
21 ○○○○
22 ○○○○
23 ○○○○
24 ○○○○
25 ○○○○
26 ○○○○

Answers and rationales

1 Correct answer—**B**

Gender identity, a conviction of being male or female, usually is established between ages 2 and 4. Once a child has become comfortable with being male or female, identification with the parent of the same sex occurs. Gender identity typically follows a patterned sequence of events. First, the sex chromosomes and gonads initiate differentiation of the reproductive anatomy; next, these visible differences act as a stimulus to parents and others to respond to the child in a manner that shapes the child's gender identity; and last, hormonal changes during adolescence activate reproductive capacity, thereby confirming the child's gender.

2 Correct answer—**B**

Follicle-stimulating hormone (FSH), combined with thyroid-stimulating hormone and an appropriate thermal environment, promotes maturation of spermatozoa. Testosterone production is stimulated by luteinizing hormone (LH), which in males is commonly referred to as interstitial cell-stimulating hormone (ICSH). High levels of testosterone, the primary male sex hormone, inhibit LH-ICSH production via pituitary function. The feedback mechanism for regulating FSH has not yet been determined. FSH does not promote production of spermatozoa or semen.

3 Correct answer—**B**

In boys, pubic hair begins to grow at the base of the penis and eventually covers the entire pubic region. The inguinal area, which contains lymphatic glands, usually is not covered with pubic hair.

4 Correct answer—**D**

Cryptorchidism, which is characterized by undescended testes, typically is detected and surgically corrected between ages 1 and 3. The testes usually descend into the scrotum during the later months of gestation. In many cases, testes that are undescended at birth descend spontaneously during the first year. If spontaneous descent does not occur, intervention at an early age prevents testicular damage caused by internal body heat and reduces the development of testicular tumors (which are more common in undescended testes). Adolescents, however, need to be examined for testicular tumors and should be taught to inspect their testes to detect abnormalities. Testicular cancer is the most common solid tumor found in males between ages 15 and 35. Testicular torsion may result from scrotal trauma; it is characterized by a testicle that hangs free from its vascular structures. Testicular inflammation is unlikely to occur in children.

5 Correct answer—C

Estrogen prevents pregnancy in several ways: It interferes with ovulation by inhibiting the release of FSH; it may inhibit the release of estrogen before ovulation and the amount of progesterone secreted after ovulation; and it may decrease the midcycle peak of LH.

6 Correct answer—B

The nurse is responsible for teaching patients about the possible health risks associated with all prescribed medications and treatments, including contraceptives. When advising Rory, the nurse should remain nonjudgmental and refrain from discussing personal values about abstinence or the value of parent-child communication. The choice of a particular method of birth control depends on the patient's preference and life-style needs. The nurse should not recommend an intrauterine device (IUD) because the incidence of pelvic inflammatory disease in adolescents who use an IUD is 5 to 10 times greater than that in adults. An infection of the reproductive organs could result in sterility.

7 Correct answer—D

Combination-type oral contraceptives are extremely reliable when taken exactly as directed, with a failure rate of less than 1%.

8 Correct answer—A

Women who use a combination-type oral contraceptive are at higher risk for hypertension than those who do not. Hypertension is defined as blood pressure greater than 140/90 mm Hg. Moderate hypertension (systolic pressure greater than 200 mm Hg; diastolic pressure between 115 and 139 mm Hg) or severe hypertension (systolic pressure between 200 and 250 mm Hg; diastolic pressure around 130 mm Hg) contraindicates the use of this medication. Chronic otitis media (ear infection), idiopathic scoliosis (curvature of the spine), and Hansen's disease (leprosy) are not contraindications.

9 Correct answer—B

A patient who misses one dose of an oral contraceptive should take that dose as soon as she remembers, then take the next dose at the regularly scheduled time. This is the best way to ensure appropriate hormonal levels on a continuous basis.

10 Correct answer—D

Marital discord has been identified as a principal factor in sexual abuse. An incestuous relationship between a parent and child typically develops in dysfunctional families in which the husband and wife no longer engage in sex. In many cases, the other parent is aware of the sexual abuse but does not intervene. Race, social status, and ethnic background have not been shown to correlate with this problem.

11 Correct answer—A

Genital herpes is a sexually transmitted disease caused by *Herpesvirus hominis*. Small, painful, vesicular lesions on the genitals, buttocks, and thighs are the primary clinical manifestation of genital herpes. Other symptoms include itching, vaginal discharge, fever, malaise, and inguinal lymphadenopathy. Macular lesions and vaginal bleeding may be associated with concurrent infection or trauma. Vaginal discharge resembling cottage cheese is associated with candidal infection.

12 Correct answer—D

No specific treatment can cure genital herpes permanently; the condition is not self-limiting. Acyclovir (Zovirax) has been used, primarily in adults, to treat the initial infection. This drug works by inhibiting viral replication; it also may shorten the symptomatic duration of acute episodes and decrease pain. However, it does not prevent recurrence or produce a permanent cure. Local application of viscous lidocaine (Xylocaine) can alleviate pain and discomfort. Penicillin, an antibiotic, would be inappropriate to treat this viral infection. Although cryotherapy can destroy the herpes lesions, it cannot remove the virus from the body.

13 Correct answer—D

The color, consistency, and odor of a vaginal discharge can help diagnose a vaginal infection. Because various infections produce different types of discharge, identifying these characteristics helps determine the diagnosis and necessary treatment. Specifically, candidiasis is associated with a thick, white, curdy discharge; gonorrhea, with a purulent, greenish-yellow discharge; *Gardnerella,* with a thin, yellow-gray, "fishy" discharge; and *Chlamydia,* with a thin or purulent discharge.

14 Correct answer—B

Although medication use, psychosocial development, and family history provide useful information, physical development is an essential component of a sexual nursing history. Assessment of physical development in female adolescents includes development of secondary sex characteristics (breast development, appearance and distribution of axillary and pubic hair) and the onset of menses. A menstrual history, which includes age of onset, frequency of periods, and amount and date of last menstrual period, also provides valuable data. Other components of a sexual history include sexual activity, contraceptive use, pregnancies, abortions, infections, and sexually transmitted diseases. Assessment of medication use may be appropriate if the adolescent has a positive history of sexually transmitted diseases or other infections (antibiotic therapy and oral contraceptives can cause candidal infections). Assessment of psychosocial development can elicit information pertaining to peer group interactions, relationships with sex partners, and body image. A family history provides information that may be helpful in circumstances in which abuse is suspected.

15 Correct answer—C

Finding out whether Sharon's boyfriend has the same symptoms will help to determine if Sharon has a sexually transmitted disease; it also will determine whether her boyfriend requires treatment. Contraception is not a means of preventing sexually transmitted diseases; therefore, assuming that the couple is not using a contraceptive method is inappropriate. Condoms may afford some protection against sexually transmitted diseases by acting as a mechanical barrier, but they should not be considered a reliable means of disease prevention. The parents' knowledge of the relationship is not the primary concern at this time. However, the nurse should consider this issue when planning the adolescent's treatment and contraceptive method.

16 Correct answer—B

Many adolescents believe that they cannot become pregnant ("It won't happen to me") and therefore do not use birth control. Also, many adolescents do not believe that they will have intercourse on a regular basis and therefore do not use a contraceptive even when one is available. By midadolescence, most girls know about reproductive physiology and how to prevent pregnancy. Although some adolescents do not use contraception because they do not want their parents to know that they are sexually active or because they prefer spontaneous sex, these reasons are not the most common responses given.

17 Correct answer—C

Tetracycline is the drug of choice for *Chlamydia* infection because of its broad spectrum of activity, which includes the chlamydial organism. However, this medication is inactive against fungi and viruses. Oral tetracycline's absorption is diminished by food and milk; I.M. injections also are poorly absorbed. Side effects include nausea, vomiting, diarrhea, anorexia, flatulence, and photosensitivity. Penicillin and its derivatives (such as amoxicillin) are ineffective against *Chlamydia*. Ceftriaxone is a cephalosporin that is structurally and pharmacologically related to penicillin and therefore also is ineffective.

18 Correct answer—B

Pneumonia is not associated with sexually transmitted diseases. Ectopic pregnancies are a common complication of sexually transmitted diseases because these diseases can damage the reproductive organs. Urinary tract infections and sepsis can result from gonorrheal infection.

19 Correct answer—A

The date of the last menstrual period may lead to a definitive diagnosis in a 15-year-old with vomiting and few, if any, other gastrointestinal symptoms. The menstrual history, a critical part of any health history, should include data about the normalcy of the last period. Although irregular cycles are common, particularly in younger teenagers, pregnancy should always be suspected, whether or not the adolescent admits to being sexually active. Information about Laura's sexual and dietary history and the time of day vomiting occurs would be more important after the pregnancy is confirmed.

20 Correct answer—C

To avoid inaccuracies and protect confidentiality, the adolescent's history must be taken in private. This is not always easy; the best approach is to ask the parent to leave the room while the patient is being examined. Parents can be told that this will help the adolescent develop a sense of responsibility for her health care. The presence of parents, siblings, or adult authority figures places pressure on the adolescent, inviting partial truths and the withholding of important information. Health history questionnaires are a quick way to conduct an interview when obtaining confidential information but may be inappropriate in an acute care setting.

21 Correct answer—D

When an adolescent is told that she is pregnant, her reaction will vary, depending on her stage of psychosocial development. A young adolescent (ages 11 to 14) who is pregnant typically displays denial or disbelief, feelings that sometimes persist into the last trimester. Such an adolescent may not even seek medical care until the pregnancy is advanced. An adolescent between ages 14 and 17 (midadolescence) may be fearful of the consequences of her pregnancy and express denial. An older adolescent (ages 17 to 20) is typically more objective when discussing options and making decisions about her future. In all cases, pregnant adolescents require careful follow-up to ensure that they are obtaining appropriate care.

22 Correct answer—D

The initial nursing action should be to assess June's condition—in this case, to determine her ability to recognize or accept her pregnancy. Junes's conclusion that her symptoms are the result of mononucleosis may indicate denial, which is a common response in young adolescents. Planning a diet, discussing fetal growth, and developing a schedule of clinic visits are planning and implementation activities that should follow assessment.

23 Correct answer—C

Many adolescents live only in the present and find it difficult to plan for the future because they are functioning in the concrete operational stage, which is characterized by inductive reasoning and beginning logic. Although they are moving toward the formal operational stage of cognitive development, which is characterized by deductive and abstract thinking, many adolescents are unable to make decisions or solve problems based on things that they have not experienced. The sensorimotor stage is characteristic of infancy. In this stage, the infant differentiates himself from the environment and develops a sense of cause and effect as he experiments with his developing motor capabilities. Children ages 2 to 7 are in the preoperational phase of development, which is characterized by egocentricity (the inability to put themselves in another person's place) and concrete thinking.

24 Correct answer—B

An adolescent's normal growth can be interrupted by pregnancy. Therefore, any diet plan must take into account the metabolic demands of the growing mother and her developing fetus; for example, the pregnant adolescent has an increased need for protein. A high-carbohydrate diet provides sufficient calories but little of the nutrition needed by the mother and fetus. Adolescent girls tend to have poor eating habits that are detrimental both to themselves and to the fetus. Only about 10% of girls who become pregnant are overweight.

25 Correct answer—B

Three hundred additional calories a day provide the necessary nutrition needed for fetal growth and development. Although this amount is the same for adult women and adolescents, adolescents vary significantly in their dietary needs. The best approach is an individualized diet plan based on the adolescent's current nutritional status, her growth needs, and the growth needs of her fetus.

26 Correct answer—D

Adolescents absorb less information through reading than through other methods, such as one-on-one demonstrations, support groups, and audiovisual aides.

CHAPTER 5

Nutrition and Feeding

Questions

1 A pediatric nutritional assessment encompasses all of the following *except:*

A. Dietary history
B. Physical measurements
C. 24-hour dietary recall
D. Caloric test

2 Which food is an important source of vitamin A?

A. Liver
B. Pork chops
C. Oranges
D. Apples

3 Calcium levels are highest in which food?

A. Broccoli
B. Prunes
C. Nuts
D. Papaya

4 The nurse should instruct the parents of a child with Hirschsprung's disease to include in the child's diet such low-residue foods as:

A. Bran or fruit muffins
B. Pork and brown rice
C. Spaghetti and chicken
D. Pancakes and sausage

5 Which breakfast foods should a child with a colostomy be encouraged to eat?

A. Raisin muffins and milk
B. Oatmeal and orange juice
C. Raw orange and banana slices and prune juice
D. Rice grain cereal and milk

6 Which of the following represents the daily caloric requirements for a 14-year-old, nonpregnant girl?

A. 2,000 kcal/day
B. 2,400 kcal/day
C. 2,800 kcal/day
D. 3,000 kcal/day

SITUATION

Cathy, age 20, recently delivered a 5³/₄ lb (2,600 g), 20" (50 cm) girl by cesarean section. Cathy participates in the Special Supplemental Food Program for Women, Infants, and Children (WIC Program) and receives food stamps; she has expressed a desire for follow-up care in the outpatient clinic. She mentions to the nurse that she has several feeding-related questions.

Questions 7 to 11 refer to this situation.

7 Cathy demonstrates her understanding of infant nutritional needs by stating that she plans to provide her child with:

A. Cow's milk beginning at age 4 months
B. Skim milk as a primary beverage
C. Evaporated milk formula
D. Ready-to-feed formula and fluoride supplements

8 Cathy demonstrates adequate feeding skills when she:

A. Judges feeding success by her infant's sleeping behavior
B. Mixes solid foods with liquids in her infant's bottle
C. Evaluates her infant's comfort level before initiating feedings
D. Allows the infant to take a bottle to bed

9 The best way for Cathy to assess the adequacy of her infant's feedings is by noting:

A. The amount of formula consumed
B. The infant's steady weight gain
C. The infant's growth rate, activity level, and general state of health
D. The infant's response to the feeding method used

SITUATION

Mrs. Murray arrives at the well-child clinic with her 11-month-old daughter, Melissa. A 24-hour dietary recall reveals that Melissa has ingested 30 oz (about 890 ml) of cow's milk, vanilla wafers, saltine crackers, one biscuit, gravy, one fried egg, 8 oz (240 ml) of fruit drink, chicken, and french fries. Melissa's hematocrit is 32%. The physician diagnoses iron-deficiency anemia.

Questions 10 and 11 refer to this situation.

10 Which sign is associated with iron-deficiency anemia in infants?

A. Constipation
B. Listlessness
C. Pallor
D. All of the above

11 Nutritional counseling for Mrs. Murray should include instructions on offering Melissa appropriate iron-rich foods, such as:

A. Iron-fortified formula, orange juice, rice cereal, egg yolks, raisins, and spinach
B. Yogurt, carrots, apple dessert, vegetables, and ham
C. Popcorn, celery sticks, chicken, and corn
D. Enriched bread, squash, bananas, and cottage cheese

SITUATION

Bud, age 10, complains of dyspnea on exertion and chest pressure when lying down at night. A medical history reveals that he dislikes gym classes and spends most of his spare time playing computer games and watching television. Physical examination reveals that he is normal except for his weight, which is 50 lb (23 kg) above the ideal weight for his age. The nurse helps Bud to develop a weight-loss program.

Questions 12 and 13 refer to this situation.

12 Exercise is an important part of any sensible weight-loss program. The best choices for Bud include:

A. Weight lifting, swimming, and baseball
B. Tennis, jogging, and weight lifting
C. Walking, tennis, golf, and swimming
D. Walking, swimming, and biking

13 Based on the available information, which nursing diagnosis is most appropriate for Bud?

A. Sleep pattern disturbance related to chest pressure when lying down at night
B. Ineffective breathing pattern related to asthma
C. Activity intolerance related to sedentary life-style and obesity
D. Pain related to unknown etiology

SITUATION

Mark Foster, a 10-month-old infant with a cleft lip and palate, is admitted to the pediatric unit for the first stage of surgical correction on his lip. Primarily breast-fed, he occasionally receives a supplemental bottle.

Questions 14 to 18 refer to this situation.

14 Feeding an infant with a cleft lip or palate offers a special challenge to the nurse because:

A. Bottle-feeding disrupts the maternal-infant bond
B. The infant has difficulty maintaining suction around a nipple
C. The nurse must discourage the infant from trying to suck
D. The infant has no desire to suck

15 Immediate postoperative complications for Mark may include:

A. Hemorrhage and respiratory distress
B. Fever and coagulation difficulties
C. Infection and hemorrhage
D. Irritability and difficulty swallowing

16 The physician orders elbow restraints postoperatively. The nurse should:

A. Put the restraints on Mark's dominant hand
B. Use the restraints only when Mark is awake
C. Use the restraints only when Mark is asleep
D. Release the restraints every 2 to 4 hours

17 Mrs. Foster is concerned about Mark's dental development. The nurse knows that an infant's first teeth, which usually erupt between ages 6 and 8 months, are the:

A. Upper lateral incisors
B. Lower central incisors
C. Lower lateral incisors
D. Upper central incisors

18 After cleft palate repair, Mark should be fed with:

A. A soup spoon
B. A dessert fork
C. A plastic syringe
D. An infant spoon

SITUATION

Mrs. Smith reveals to the visiting nurse that Nicholas, age 2 weeks, has been vomiting about 3 tablespoons of previously ingested food daily for the past 3 days. The vomitus contains no blood or bile. Mrs. Smith tells the nurse that she feeds Nicholas 4 oz (120 ml) of a soy-based, iron-fortified formula (Similac 20 with Iron) every 4 hours and that the vomiting occurs effortlessly regardless of the neonate's position. Nicholas's growth parameters have remained unchanged since birth. The physician suspects gastroesophageal reflux.

Questions 19 and 20 refer to this situation.

19 To prevent Nicholas from aspirating during or after a feeding, Mrs. Smith should:

A. Keep Nicholas prone at a 15-degree angle after feeding
B. Thicken the morning and evening feedings with cereal
C. Administer large-volume feedings every 6 hours
D. Maintain Nicholas in an upright position, at a 60-degree angle, without an infant seat

20 To evaluate the effectiveness of Nicholas's home care program, the nurse should consider which of the following as most important?

A. Absence of spitting up
B. Weight gain
C. Ability to tolerate clear liquids between feedings
D. Tolerance of feedings scheduled every 6 hours

SITUATION

Jennifer, a full-term neonate, is transferred to the neonatal intensive care unit after X-rays reveal that her esophagus ends in a blind pouch. She has had problems with feeding and is now on nothing-by-mouth (NPO) status. Her diagnosis is esophageal atresia; surgery is scheduled for the next morning.

Questions 21 to 24 refer to this situation.

21 Which physical findings are commonly associated with esophageal atresia?

A. Decreased bowel sounds
B. Choking, coughing, and cyanosis
C. Visible gastric peristaltic waves
D. Jaundice and drooling

22 Which position is best for Jennifer preoperatively?

A. Prone on her abdomen
B. Right side-lying
C. Supine, with her head and chest elevated 30 degrees
D. Left side-lying

23 To prevent aspiration of secretions, the nurse must suction Jennifer every 2 to 4 hours as needed. Prolonged and vigorous suctioning of a neonate can cause:

A. Pallor
B. Tachycardia
C. Laryngospasm
D. Pneumonia

24 Jennifer has a gastrostomy tube in place postoperatively. The nurse must unclamp the tube and attach it to a syringe for ½ hour after each feeding. This procedure is necessary for all of the following reasons *except:*

A. It acts as a safety valve when vomiting occurs
B. It facilitates the next feeding
C. It allows for reflux of air and gastric contents when the neonate cries
D. It prevents pressure on the suture line

SITUATION

Ms. Thompson arrives at the emergency department with Josh, her 7-month-old son, whom she describes as being colicky and irritable during the past 3 weeks. She tells the nurse that Josh has lost weight over the past 3 months. Josh is suspected of having celiac disease and is hospitalized for testing and evaluation.

Questions 25 to 27 refer to this situation.

25 The stools of a patient with celiac disease are characteristically:

A. Steatorrhic
B. Tarry
C. Bloody
D. Putty-colored

26 Celiac disease involves an intolerance of:

A. Phenylalanine
B. Glucose
C. Gluten
D. Triglycerides

27 Which food should be eliminated from the Josh's diet?

A. Strained peas
B. Soy-based infant formula
C. Creamed corn
D. Strained spaghetti

SITUATION

Shari, age 17, was admitted to the hospital 2 days ago for dehydration and hypokalemia. On admission, she said that she had the flu for a few days. Last evening, she was found sitting on the bathroom floor, crying because she feared that the I.V. fluid she was receiving would make her fat and ugly. She is 5'4" (163 cm) tall and weighs 123 lb (56 kg). Her weight has fluctuated by 20 lb (9 kg) over the past year.

Questions 28 to 33 refer to this situation.

---

28 Which assessment finding is the most reliable indication of an eating disorder in this patient?

A. Dehydration
B. Hypokalemia
C. Crying about body image
D. Frequent weight fluctuations

---

29 Which statement most accurately describes bulimia nervosa?

A. Intense aversion to food and weight gain
B. Recurrent episodes of binge eating, followed by extreme measures to prevent weight gain
C. Deliberate starvation by self-induced vomiting
D. Intermittent weight control by self-induced vomiting

---

30 Which physical finding is *not* associated with self-induced vomiting?

A. Russell's sign
B. Enlarged parotid glands
C. Elevated amylase level
D. Amenorrhea

---

31 When a bulimic patient exhibits signs of depression, the nurse's priority is to:

A. Assess for suicidal tendencies
B. Promote healthy self-esteem
C. Encourage peer interaction
D. Monitor sleeping patterns

32 How long after meals should the nurse observe a bulimic patient for self-induced vomiting?

A. ½ hour
B. 1 hour
C. 2 hours
D. 4 hours

33 Shari has a history of wine and cheese binges. Which antidepressant should *not* be prescribed?

A. Imipramine (Tofranil)
B. Amitryptyline (Elavil)
C. Trazodone (Desyrel)
D. Phenelzine (Nardil)

SITUATION

Karen, age 14, is admitted to the hospital for the fourth time for bradycardia and hypotension secondary to anorexia nervosa. Anorexic for the past 2 years, Karen is 5′ (152 cm) tall and weighs 68 lb (31 kg). She has a history of multiple food-related behaviors and exercises for 3 hours every day.

Questions 34 to 38 refer to this situation.

34 Which statement best describes the disorted body image of a patient with anorexia nervosa?

A. The severity of the distortion depends on the amount of the weight loss
B. The distortion is transient and appears only when the patient is 15% below her expected body weight
C. The distortion is present even when the patient's weight is normal
D. The distortion involves feeling fat even when emaciated, or believing that a specific area of the body is too fat

35 Anorexia nervosa is caused by:

A. Faulty development of selfhood
B. Malfunctioning hypothalamus
C. Dysfunctional family dynamics
D. Many unknown factors

36 The nurse should suspect anorexia nervosa in a patient with significant weight loss and:

A. Amenorrhea, diarrhea, and decreased urine output
B. Amenorrhea, constipation, and hypotension
C. Amenorrhea, tachycardia, and diarrhea
D. Amenorrhea, constipation, and decreased urine output

37 When providing care, the nurse should be concerned with Karen's:

A. Appetite development
B. Fixation on calorie counting
C. Normalization of eating behaviors
D. Rapid weight gain

38 When planning an exercise regimen for Karen, the nurse should:

A. Avoid any exercise-related discussions with the patient
B. Discourage the patient from exercising
C. Stress the importance of exercise as a means of promoting fitness
D. Discourage the patient from performing aerobic exercises

SITUATION

Linda, who was born at 34 weeks' gestation, is in a level-III intensive care nursery where she is being fed every 2 hours with gavage feedings.

Questions 39 to 41 refer to this situation.

39 Frequent removal and insertion of a gavage feeding tube can result in which complication?

A. Increased gastric emptying
B. Physiologic anemia
C. Vagal stimulation
D. Hemoconcentration

40 Which finding suggests that Linda cannot tolerate intermittent gavage feedings?

   A. Delayed gastric emptying
   B. Absence of apneic and bradycardic episodes
   C. Aspiration of 1 ml of gastric contents before each feeding
   D. Increased tolerance for larger volumes of food

41 Some formulas for premature infants are whey-based because:

   A. They contain more casein than non-whey-based formulas
   B. They contain more iron than non-whey-based formulas
   C. Premature infants have a decreased ability to digest casein
   D. Premature infants have a decreased need for protein

Answer sheet

	A	B	C	D			A	B	C	D
1	○	○	○	○		31	○	○	○	○
2	○	○	○	○		32	○	○	○	○
3	○	○	○	○		33	○	○	○	○
4	○	○	○	○		34	○	○	○	○
5	○	○	○	○		35	○	○	○	○
6	○	○	○	○		36	○	○	○	○
7	○	○	○	○		37	○	○	○	○
8	○	○	○	○		38	○	○	○	○
9	○	○	○	○		39	○	○	○	○
10	○	○	○	○		40	○	○	○	○
11	○	○	○	○		41	○	○	○	○
12	○	○	○	○						
13	○	○	○	○						
14	○	○	○	○						
15	○	○	○	○						
16	○	○	○	○						
17	○	○	○	○						
18	○	○	○	○						
19	○	○	○	○						
20	○	○	○	○						
21	○	○	○	○						
22	○	○	○	○						
23	○	○	○	○						
24	○	○	○	○						
25	○	○	○	○						
26	○	○	○	○						
27	○	○	○	○						
28	○	○	○	○						
29	○	○	○	○						
30	○	○	○	○						

Answers and rationales

1 Correct answer—**D**

A caloric test is not related to nutritional assessment. This test, which is used in neurologic examinations for children with central nervous system disorders, involves irrigating the external auditory canal with ice water and observing eye movement. The dietary history is an important element in all pediatric nutritional assessments. The nurse asks the parent or child questions about a variety of behaviors, including eating habits, appetite, food preferences and dislikes, food preparation, cultural influences, feeding difficulties, special diets, and diet supplements. Physical measurements that pertain to nutritional status include height, weight, head and arm circumference, and skinfold thickness. A dietary recall, in which the parent records all intake for a 24-hour period, is commonly obtained to assess a child's food intake. The amount and type of calories consumed can be evaluated from this information.

2 Correct answer—**A**

Vitamin A is found in some animal sources, such as liver, kidney, milk and milk products, fish oil, and egg yolk. Other significant sources of vitamin A are yellow and green fruits and vegetables (such as carrots, sweet potatoes, squash, apricots, spinach, collards, broccoli, and cabbage). This vitamin helps to maintain healthy skin and mucous membranes and increases the body's resistance to infection. Additionally, vitamin A plays a critical role in the eye's ability to adapt to light and darkness. Insufficient amounts of vitamin A in the retina can cause night blindness. Children require 400 to 700 mg of vitamin A daily.

3 Correct answer—**A**

Calcium levels are highest in broccoli, kale, and mustard and turnip greens, as well as in dairy products, sardines, and salmon bones. Calcium is essential for bone growth and development, blood clotting, and neuromuscular function. Children need about 800 mg of calcium daily.

4 Correct answer—**C**

Spaghetti and chicken should be included in the diet of a child with Hirshsprung's disease—a congenital disorder in which parasympathetic innervation to an area of the colon is absent, resulting in the absence of peristalsis in this area, accumulation of bowel contents, and increased risk of bowel obstruction. Children with Hirschsprung's disease require a low-residue diet to decrease the bulk of the bowel contents and minimize bowel irritation. Children generally enjoy low-residue foods, such as spaghetti, lean broiled hamburgers on white bread, broiled chicken, vanilla or chocolate ice cream, crackers, plain cookies, and gelatin desserts.

5 Correct answer—D

The diet for a child with a colostomy should be high-calorie and low-residue for easy evacuation. Rice grain cereal and milk are both low-residue foods. High-residue foods include raw fruits, such as raisins and oranges, and oatmeal.

6 Correct answer—B

About 2,400 calories provide adequate energy for a nonpregnant 14-year-old girl's growth and development.

7 Correct answer—D

Commercially prepared ready-to-feed formulas are appropriate nutritional sources for infants. However, because these formulas are premixed, fluoridated tap water is not added to the preparation and fluoride supplements are necessary. Because cow's milk contains minute amounts of essential fatty acids, it usually is not recommended during the first year. Drinking skim milk forces infants to use their own body fat for energy. Although evaporated milk formula is an appropriate nutritional source, it must be accompanied by supplements of iron, vitamin C, and fluoride (if the water supply is not fluoridated).

8 Correct answer—C

Caregivers should evaluate their infant's behavior before feedings. In this way, they can become adept at recognizing cues and patterns of hunger. No correlation has been found between ingestion of food and sleeping behavior. Solid foods should not be mixed with liquids and fed through the nipple of an infant's bottle. The purpose of introducing solid foods is to allow the infant to experience different textures and modes of ingestion; mixing solids with liquids in a bottle does not encourage the infant to experience new sensations. Allowing an infant to take a bottle to bed is unwise because it may lead to tooth decay.

9 Correct answer—**C**

Determining whether an infant is receiving adequate nutrition is based on observing growth rate, activity level, and state of health. The infant should demonstrate growth (increased height, weight, and head circumference) within the parameters for her age. She also should have enough energy to sustain physical activity and achieve developmental milestones. A general state of health that is free of physiological imbalances and disorders reflects adequate nutritional intake. The amount of formula consumed or weight gain alone do not determine the adequacy of feedings. Regardless of feeding method, an infant's weight gain should be balanced in relation to her height and age.

10 Correct answer—**D**

Anemia—a decrease in hemoglobin below normal levels (9 to 14 g/dl at age 2 months)—results in the decreased ability of blood to carry oxygen to the tissues. Anemia that develops slowly may cause no noticeable symptoms. However, infants with severe anemia may suffer from constipation, pallor, listlessness, and loss of appetite. If the anemia is untreated, tissue hypoxia can result, as evidenced by muscle weakness, fatigue, and altered functioning of the cardiovascular and central nervous systems. Infants with iron-deficiency anemia are treated with oral or injectable iron supplements.

11 Correct answer—**A**

Egg yolks, spinach, raisins, rice cereal, and iron-fortified formula are good sources of iron for an 11-month-old infant. Orange juice is an excellent source of vitamin C, which helps to improve iron absorption. The other foods are poor sources of iron, providing small amounts at best. Popcorn and celery are inappropriate foods for an 11-month-old, who may choke on them.

12 Correct answer—**D**

Because they increase energy expenditure, aerobic exercises are more effective than anaerobic exercises in a weight-loss program. Walking, swimming, and biking can be performed at increasing levels of intensity and duration as Bud's exercise tolerance increases. Bud can also continue these activities as he grows older. Bud can walk, swim, or bike in a group or by himself, and the related costs are not prohibitive. Weight lifting, baseball, tennis, and golf are not aerobic exercises. Baseball and tennis require participation by other individuals, and cost may be a deterrent for activities such as golf, tennis, and weightlifting.

13 Correct answer—C

Fat deposits in the thoracic and abdominal walls interfere with movement of the diaphragm and accessory respiratory muscles, thereby decreasing a person's ability to expand intrathoracically during inspiration. Sleeping horizontally increases the pressure of these abdominal and thoracic fat deposits against the diaphragm and accessory muscles. Fat cells also increase the body's oxygen demands, especially during exertion. This supports the nursing diagnosis of *Activity intolerance related to sedentary life-style and obesity.* Although Bud reported chest pressure when lying down at night, he did not mention that his sleep was disturbed or that he was in pain. Asthma is not a factor in this situation because the physical examination findings were normal.

14 Correct answer—B

Feeding an infant with a cleft lip or palate is difficult because the infant has trouble maintaining suction around a nipple. This in turn interferes with his ability to suck. An infant's desire to suck is strong, and one with a cleft lip or palate is no exception. Sucking motions should be encouraged because they promote the development of muscles that later will play a role in speech development. The maternal-infant bond is not affected by bottle feeding.

15 Correct answer—A

Respiratory distress commonly follows surgery to correct a cleft lip because the infant must adjust to breathing through his nose instead of through the now-closed cleft. Postsurgical edema and increased secretions also may cause respiratory distress, and the highly vascular facial area is subject to bleeding. Fever and infection may occur later. Coagulation difficulties are not associated with cleft lip and palate repair as long as the coagulation studies were normal before the surgery. The child is likely to be irritable from discomfort, restricted positioning, and elbow restraints, but this is not a complication. Difficulty swallowing is an expected result of the surgery, because of discomfort, breathing through the nose, and drainage of secretions.

16 Correct answer—**D**

Elbow restraints prevent an infant from touching the postoperative site, where he could rub or disturb the suture line. The restraints should be placed on both hands in the postoperative period and should remain in place whether the infant is asleep or awake. The elbow restraints should be removed every 2 to 4 hours to exercise the infant's arms, provide relief from restrictions, and observe for signs of skin breakdown. The nurse should release one restraint at a time, especially if the infant is very active. The parents should continue to use the restraints on discharge until the suture line is well healed.

17 Correct answer—**B**

The lower central incisors are commonly the first teeth to erupt, usually between ages 6 and 8 months. The other teeth typically erupt as follows: upper central incisors, 8 to 12 months; upper lateral incisors, 9 to 13 months; lower lateral incisors, 10 to 16 months; upper first molars, 13 to 19 months; lower first molars, 14 to 18 months; upper cuspids, 16 to 22 months; lower cuspids, 17 to 23 months; lower second molars, 23 to 31 months; and upper second molars, 25 to 33 months.

18 Correct answer—**A**

A child with a repaired cleft palate may be fed carefully with a soup spoon or from the side of a regular spoon. Use of a large-bowled spoon prevents the utensil from being inserted into the mouth, where it could injure the suture line.

19 Correct answer—**D**

When an infant is seated upright at a 60-degree angle, food is kept down by gravity. Gravity also may prevent gastroesophageal reflux (GER) and help clear refluxed material from the esophagus. An infant younger than age 6 months tends to slump when placed in an infant seat; such a position will increase abdominal pressure, predisposing him to GER. Some research suggests that an infant age 6 months or younger may benefit by remaining in a prone position at 30 degrees for 24 hours a day. An infant with GER whose growth is not adversely affected requires no intervention; he probably will outgrow the disorder. Intervention for a symptomatic infant with GER involves giving small, thickened feedings every 2 to 3 hours and placing him upright at a 60-degree angle. Decreased vomiting usually occurs within 2 weeks with such a regimen. However, even though thickened feedings may help to prevent reflux, they will not keep the infant from aspirating refluxed food. If the GER is severe, pharmacologic intervention with drugs that enhance gastric emptying may be necessary. Surgery may be indicated for infants who develop complications, such as respiratory distress, esophagitis, or esophageal stricture.

20 Correct answer—B

Weight gain is the most important parameter when assessing an infant's feeding tolerance. A small amount of spitting up may continue for a few weeks. The infant should receive small-volume feedings thickened with cereal every 2 to 3 hours for up to 6 weeks. If the infant does not gain weight and continues to spit up, surgery may be indicated.

21 Correct answer—B

Esophageal atresia is a congenital anomaly in which the esophagus ends in a blind pouch instead of forming a continuous passage to the stomach. This abnormality is suspected in a neonate with excessive salivation and drooling accompanied by choking, coughing, and sneezing. When Jennifer is fed, she swallows normally, then coughs and struggles. The food then returns through her nose and mouth. A neonate can become cyanotic and may stop breathing as the overflow of fluid from the blind pouch is aspirated into the trachea and bronchi.

22 Correct answer—C

The best position for a neonate with esophageal atresia is supine, with the head of the bed elevated at least 30 degrees. This position minimizes the reflux of gastric secretions.

23 Correct answer—C

A neonate's larynx is structurally different from that of an adult. Because the cartilage of a neonate's larynx is soft and pliable, laryngospasm can occur during suctioning. This complication can lead to hypoxemia and pallor. Tachycardia and pneumonia are not associated with suctioning.

24 Correct answer—**B**

A gastrostomy is a common component of the surgical management of a gastrointestinal disease. It provides a means for early postoperative nutrition and gastric decompression. Usually the gastrostomy tube is left open to provide a safety valve during vomiting, to allow for reflux of air and gastric contents during crying, and to prevent pressure on the suture line. The syringe should not be left in place until the next feeding because the neonate's mobility is restricted when the tube is unclamped.

25 Correct answer—**A**

Celiac disease causes changes in the intestinal mucosa that reduce fat absorption. Steatorrhea is defined as foul, frothy, fatty, greasy-looking stools. This condition is typical in diseases involving malabsorption of fat from the bowel. Tarry, bloody, or putty-colored stools are not associated with this disease.

26 Correct answer—**C**

Celiac disease is sometimes called celiac sprue, nontropical sprue, or gluten-induced enteropathy. This condition is a permanent intolerance to the protein gluten, which is found in rye, wheat, barley, and oat products. Whether celiac disease is a genetic disorder, an inborn metabolic disorder, or an immunologic disorder is not known.

27 Correct answer—**D**

Celiac disease is primarily treated through dietary restriction. Vitamin supplementation and parenteral nutrition may be indicated if the child is extremely malnourished. Dietary management of this disease is accomplished by eliminating foods that contain wheat, rye, barley, or oats. Maintaining such a regimen usually is difficult; aside from the obvious food sources, other prepared foods may contain the prohibited grains (for example, gluten may be listed as "hydrolyzed vegetable protein" on some food labels). Many forbidden foods are favorites of children (such as pizza, hot dogs, cake, doughnuts, and candy). Spaghetti is made from wheat flour, which contains gluten. Children with celiac disease usually can tolerate soy-based products, peas, and corn. Other acceptable foods that appeal to children are applesauce, cooked fruit, bananas, eggs, cheese, and gelatin desserts.

28 Correct answer—C

A persistent and unrealistic concern about body image is characteristic of a person with an eating disorder. Shari demonstrates a distorted body image by believing that the I.V. fluid will make her
fat. Although dehydration, hypokalemia, and weight fluctuations
may be associated with an eating disorder, they are not the most reliable indicators of this problem. Dehydration and hypokalemia
may be signs of other illnesses, such as a gastrointestinal virus or
an endocrine dysfunction. Weight fluctuations are not universal to
all eating disorders.

29 Correct answer—B

Binging is the classic symptom of bulimia nervosa. It occurs in recurrent episodes, followed by fasting, self-induced vomiting, laxative abuse, diuretic abuse, or vigorous exercise. Although the bulimic patient has an aversion to weight gain, she usually has no
aversion to food. However, she may avoid specific foods. A bulimic patient uses self-induced vomiting to prevent weight gain, not
to induce starvation. The last option is incorrect because it does
not mention binging, a primary component of the bulimic patient's
binge-purge cycle.

30 Correct answer—D

Amenorrhea can be associated with eating disorders, but it is not a
symptom of self-induced vomiting. Russell's sign is a bruise or
scarring noted at the base of the index finger; it results from abrasion when a person continually forces her finger down her throat.
The parotid glands may enlarge because of the constant acid bath
from gastric secretions. This irritation also may result in an elevated amylase level.

31 Correct answer—A

Depression always warrants an assessment for suicidal tendencies.
Bulimic patients are prone to depression, and suicide is a common
cause of death in this group. When dealing with such patients, the
nurse should suspect depression and assess for suicidal ideation.
The nurse can promote healthy self-esteem and encourage peer interaction in an attempt to relieve the depression; however, these actions are not priorities. Changes in sleeping patterns may indicate

depression, but monitoring sleeping behavior is not a primary concern.

32 Correct answer—C

Eating disorders can delay gastric emptying for up to 2 hours. Therefore, the nurse must observe the patient for this length of time to prevent her from vomiting the contents of her meal.

33 Correct answer—D

Eating foods with a high tyramine content, such as aged cheeses, wine, beer, yogurt, and yeast extract, and taking diet pills can produce a hypertensive crisis in a patient receiving a monoamine oxidase (MAO) inhibitor, such as phenelzine (Nardil). Hypertensive crisis, which is characterized by intense occipital headache, palpitations, marked hypertension, sweating, nausea, vomiting, chest pain, bradycardia or tachycardia, fever, stiff neck, photophobia, and intracranial bleeding, can be fatal. Impipramine (Tofranil), amitryptyline (Elavil), and trazodone (Desyrel) are not MAO inhibitors and do not have these dietary restrictions.

34 Correct answer—D

An anorectic patient such as Karen feels fat even when she is extremely emaciated. She also may believe that specific body parts, such as her thighs, hips, buttocks, and abdomen, are fat even though they are not. The key term in anorexia nervosa is distortion. The severity of the distortion is unrelated to the patient's weight.

35 Correct answer—D

Although several theories exist, the etiology of anorexia nervosa remains unknown. Many theorists and practitioners believe that anorexia nervosa is a multifactorial disorder, involving the individual, her family, and her culture. An anorectic patient typically is a member of a disorganized family that is riddled with conflict; thus the patient may be using food to gain control over one aspect of her life. Anorexia nervosa may be caused by a biochemical abnormality. Many individuals with this disorder stop menstruating before the onset of anorexia nervosa, indicating that a hypothalamus malfunction may be involved. Genetics also may play a role—more than 90% of persons with anorexia nervosa are female.

36 Correct answer—B

Amenorrhea, constipation, and hypotension result from starvation-induced weight loss. Diarrhea is not a common symptom of anorexia nervosa. Tachycardia also is not a symptom, although it may accompany dehydration. Increased, not decreased, urine output is a common finding. In some patients, the kidneys have difficulty concentrating urine in response to water deprivation; this may result from defective osmoregulation of vasopressin secretion. (Vasopressin increases the resorption of water in the distal tubules of the kidney, thereby decreasing the amount of urine excreted.) Few patients have vasopressin responses consistent with partial diabetes insipidus.

37 Correct answer—C

A primary nursing goal in caring for an anorectic patient is the normalization of eating habits. The nurse should ensure that Karen receives three adequately spaced, nutritional meals each day and discourage bizarre food behaviors, such as hoarding (accumulating and hiding food). The term *anorexia* actually is a misnomer because an anorectic patient has an appetite over which she exhibits tremendous control. Fixation on calorie counting is an abnormal food-related behavior and should be discouraged. Rapid weight gain also should be avoided because it may cause the patient to feel out of control. It also may stress the patient's cardiovascular system, possibly leading to death (rapid weight gain is a leading cause of death in the rehabilitative stage of this disorder).

38 Correct answer—C

Exercise should be promoted as a means of improving fitness rather than appearance. Discouraging or not discussing exercise programs is inadvisable because moderate exercise can promote physical fitness and development, enhance psychological well-being, and provide opportunities for social interaction. The nurse should develop an individualized exercise program for Karen; aerobics can be included in this program.

39 Correct answer—C

Frequent insertion and removal of a gavage feeding tube is associated with stimulation of the vagus nerve (10th cranial nerve), which contains fibers that supply most of the organs of the neck, thorax, and abdomen. Vagal stimulation has an inhibitory effect on the heart and can increase the risk of apnea and bradycardia in premature neonates. Increased gastric emptying, anemia, and hemoconcentration are unrelated to gavage feeding.

40 Correct answer—A

Delayed gastric emptying is associated with an inability to tolerate intermittent gavage feedings. Obtaining a small amount (less than 2 ml) of aspirate before feedings, with a gradual increased tolerance for larger volumes of food, is an indication that the neonate is tolerating the feedings. Absence of apneic and bradycardic episodes signifies that insertion of the feeding tube is not stimulating the vagus nerve.

41 Correct answer—C

Premature infants have a decreased ability to digest casein proteins because they lack sufficient proteolytic enzymes. They are commonly given whey-based formulas because these formulas contain less casein than other formulas. Premature infants usually have an increased need for protein because protein stores are low. Whey content and iron content are unrelated.

CHAPTER 6

Allergy and Infection

Questions

1 The nurse prepares to administer penicillin V potassium (Ledercillin VK) to a child with pneumonia. Which statement about this medication is *true?*

A. It is excreted in the urine and may produce a characteristic odor
B. It is slowly absorbed from the gastrointestinal tract
C. It should be administered only if the child has a cough
D. It does not require refrigeration if it is prescribed as an oral suspension

2 The pediatrician prescribes ampicillin (Amcill) 300 mg I.V. every 12 hours for a neonate with sepsis. The medication yields 500 mg/ml when mixed with a diluent. How many milliliters should the nurse administer?

A. 0.5 ml
B. 0.6 ml
C. 1 ml
D. 6 ml

3 Which nursing action has priority when a child is diagnosed with AIDS?

A. Psychosocial support
B. Patient teaching
C. Social assessment
D. Home assessment

SITUATION

Gary Thomas, age 9 months, has been referred to an allergist for a diagnostic workup. He has a constantly runny nose, a frequent cough, and moderately severe atopic dermatitis. He is being treated for his third ear infection in 3 months.

Questions 4 to 7 refer to this situation.

4 The nurse at the allergist's office takes an extensive history. Which information elicted from Gary's parents is most significant?

A. Gary was born 2 weeks postmature and was colicky during his first 3 months
B. Mr. Thomas is allergic to penicillin, and Gary does not sleep through the night
C. Gary regurgitates his formula frequently, and Mrs. Thomas has hay fever
D. Mrs. Thomas has hay fever, and both parents smoke

5 The nurse should include which statement in her discussion of atopic dermatitis with Gary's parents?

A. Atopic dermatitis is not contagious
B. Heat and humidity exacerbate the itching
C. The lesions will not leave permanent scars
D. All of the above

6 The allergist prescribes hydrocortisone 1% (Hytone) cream for topical application twice a day to areas of atopic dermatitis. The nurse instructs Gary's parents in general skin care, cream application, and infection control measures. Which instruction is most important to stress to the parents?

A. Spread a thick film of the prescribed cream on the affected areas daily and wash the affected areas once a week
B. Gently abrade the skin before applying the cream to enhance absorption
C. Limit the use of soap and water and use an emollient cream at least 4 times a day
D. Wash the affected areas frequently and use a moisturizing cream sparingly

7 The allergist determines that Gary is allergic to cow's milk and recommends a soy-based formula instead. As Gary begins eating more solid foods, the nurse should instruct Gary's parents to:

A. Begin including dairy products in Gary's meals
B. Check food labels for the presence of casein and whey
C. Use non-fat dry milk in cooking
D. Be sure that Gary drinks extra formula

SITUATION

Max Bower, age 9, has a recent history of upper respiratory tract infections. He was just diagnosed as having rheumatic fever.

Questions 8 to 12 refer to this situation.

---

8 Rheumatic fever is commonly associated with a history of infection by which organism?

A. *Haemophilus influenzae*
B. Group A streptococcus
C. Pneumococcus
D. *Staphylococcus aureus*

---

9 Which sequela is predominant in rheumatic fever?

A. Nervous system damage
B. Joint damage
C. Heart damage
D. Subcutaneous nodule development

---

10 Diagnosis of rheumatic fever is based on modification of the Jones criteria. These criteria include evidence of all of the following *except:*

A. Major clinical manifestations, such as carditis and chorea
B. Minor clinical manifestations, such as fever and arthralgia
C. Supportive evidence, such as an elevated antistreptolysin-O titer
D. Family history of rheumatic fever in one or both parents

---

11 Which control measure is most important for preventing rheumatic fever?

A. Using a throat culture to identify and treat streptococcal infections
B. Administering prophylactic penicillin to all persons in a high-risk age-group
C. Adhering to prescribed regimens of rest and nutrition
D. Maintaining a healthy state to ward off infections

12 Nursing care for Max should include all of the following *except:*

A. Providing rest and adequate nutrition throughout the recuperation period
B. Educating him about the importance of adhering to a prescribed medication regimen
C. Isolating him to prevent disease transmission
D. Providing emotional support to him and his family

SITUATION

Stephen, age 6 months, and his sister Janie, age 4, were born to a drug-abusing mother who tested positive for the human immunodeficiency virus (HIV). The family is new to the community, and the children are enrolled in a day-care center. They are brought to the clinic with cold symptoms; their HIV status is unknown.

Questions 13 to 15 refer to this situation.

---

13 Which assessment finding leads the nurse to suspect that the children may be HIV-positive?

A. Pallor
B. Recurrent diarrhea
C. Hydrocephaly
D. Vomiting

---

14 The nurse knows that any HIV-positive child who attends a day-care center should receive which immunizations?

A. Diptheria, pertussis, tetanus (DPT) and inactivated polio virus (IPV)
B. Diptheria, pertussis, tetanus (DPT) and oral polio virus (OPV)
C. Pneumococcal and *Haemophilus influenzae* type b (Hib)
D. Measles, mumps, rubella (MMR) and immune globulin

15 If Stephen and Janie are HIV-positive, which precaution at the day-care center is necessary?

A. Having all workers wear masks and gloves when coming in contact with Stephen and Janie
B. Barring Stephen and Janie from attending the day-care center
C. Disinfecting surfaces soiled with Stephen's and Janie's blood or body fluids with a bleach solution
D. Sending a letter to the other children's parents informing them that two HIV-positive children attend the center

Answer sheet

	A	B	C	D
1	○	○	○	○
2	○	○	○	○
3	○	○	○	○
4	○	○	○	○
5	○	○	○	○
6	○	○	○	○
7	○	○	○	○
8	○	○	○	○
9	○	○	○	○
10	○	○	○	○
11	○	○	○	○
12	○	○	○	○
13	○	○	○	○
14	○	○	○	○
15	○	○	○	○

Answers and rationales

1 Correct answer—**A**

Penicillin V potassium is a bactericidal agent used for streptococcal, pneumococcal, and staphylococcal infections. It is rapidly excreted by the kidneys and produces a characteristic odor. This drug also is rapidly absorbed by the gastrointestinal tract and is best taken with food. Penicillin V potassium must be administered on a regular schedule for the prescribed number of days or until the medication is finished. Children who are asymptomatic should continue to receive the medication for the prescribed duration. Oral suspensions must be refrigerated. The nurse should shake the suspension before giving the medication to the child to ensure the correct dosage.

2 Correct answer—**B**

The neonate should receive 0.6 ml of ampicillin.
$$\frac{300 \text{ mg}}{x} = \frac{500 \text{ mg}}{1 \text{ ml}}$$
$$300 = 500x$$
$$x = 0.6 \text{ ml}$$

3 Correct answer—**A**

Psychosocial support is a vital nursing action when a child is diagnosed with AIDS. At the time of diagnosis, the parents and child typically experience denial, guilt, and anger. The nurse should help the family to accept the diagnosis to ensure that the child receives appropriate follow-up care. Psychosocial support provides opportunities for the parents and child to express their feelings and concerns. The child's family usually is too overwhelmed to comprehend any teaching at this time. Social and home assessments—which determine what support the family needs to care for the child—can be obtained after the initial shock of the diagnosis subsides; in an interdisciplinary team approach, the social worker is responsible for these assessments.

4 Correct answer—**D**

Research indicates that about 87% of all allergic children have a close relative with an allergic disorder. The risk of developing allergic rhinitis can be as high as 50% in a child whose parents have allergies. Eczema or atopic dermatitis is more common in children whose parents have hay fever or asthma. Research has shown that children of parents who smoke have more respiratory infections, hospitalizations, wheezing episodes, school absences, and diminished lung function than children whose parents do not smoke. Postmaturity is not related to allergic disorders. Gary may not sleep through the night because of his cough or pruritus associated with atopic dermatitis. Failure to sleep through the night or regurgitating formula may be symptoms of an allergic disorder but are not factors in determining Gary's susceptibility to allergies.

5 Correct answer—D

The nurse should inform the parents that atopic dermatitis is not contagious. She also should instruct them to avoid overdressing the child because heat and humidity lead to perspiration and intensified itching; lightweight and loose-fitting clothing minimizes overheating and irritation to the lesions. Parents typically are relieved to learn that the lesions do not leave permanent scars.

6 Correct answer—C

The parents should avoid washing the areas with soap and water because this removes moisture from the horny layer of the skin. Emollient creams applied in a thin layer will hold moisture in the skin, provide a barrier to environmental irritants, and prevent infection. Topical steroid creams, such as hydrocortisone 1% (Hytone), should be applied sparingly as a light film. The affected areas should be cleaned gently with water before applying the cream. Abrading the skin can increase the risk of infection and alter the absorption of medication. Excessive application of steroidal creams may result in systemic absorption and Cushing's syndrome. Frequent washing dries the skin, making it more susceptible to cracking and further breakdown.

7 Correct answer—B

Cow's milk allergy results from a sensitivity to one or more milk proteins. As the infant begins to eat more solid foods, his parents should check food labels for the presence of milk proteins, which may be listed as lactose, caseinate, sodium caseinate, lactalbumin, curds, or whey. Non-fat dry milk and other milk products contain milk proteins. As Gary's consumption of solid foods increases, his consumption of formula should decrease.

8 Correct answer—**B**

Rheumatic fever may develop 2 to 6 weeks after an infection caused by group A beta-hemolytic streptococcus. Usually, the streptococcal infection is one that affects the upper respiratory tract, such as strep throat. Rheumatic fever is not an infection but possibly an autoimmune response to the streptococcal infection. The incidence of this disease in children ages 5 to 9 is approximately 0.5 per 100,000; children who live in crowded environmental conditions are at higher risk because they are more likely to be exposed to such organisms as streptococci. Primary symptoms include an erythematous macular rash, fever, swollen and tender joints, cardiac inflammation, and central nervous system (CNS) disturbances. The CNS manifestations, known as *chorea,* include muscle weakness, speech disturbances, and involuntary movements.

9 Correct answer—**C**

Cardiac involvement is the chief cause for concern in patients with rheumatic fever. Carditis occurs in varying degrees of severity; scarring of the mitral and aortic valves and permanent damage to the heart may result. Disturbances of the CNS can be the most distressing aspect of the disease for the child, but these symptoms resolve with no permanent damage. Pathological changes in the joints—caused by edema, inflammation, and effusion into the joint tissue—occur during the first few weeks of illness, then resolve without permanent consequences. Nontender subcutaneous nodes may persist for some time, then disappear gradually and spontaneously.

10 Correct answer—**D**

Jones criteria include evidence of major manifestations of the disease (cardiac, joint, skin, and CNS disturbances); minor manifestations of the disease (fever, epistaxis, abdominal pain, arthralgia, weakness, fatigue, pallor, anorexia, and weight loss); laboratory findings (increased erythrocyte sedimentation rate and leukocyte count); and supportive findings (positive throat culture for streptococci and an elevated or increasing antistreptolysin-O titer). There is no evidence that the disease is transmitted genetically.

11 Correct answer—A

Identifying a streptococcal infection by a throat culture and promptly treating it with an antibiotic is the best way to prevent rheumatic fever. Rheumatic fever occurs primarily in school-age children; however, administering prophylactic antibiotics to all children in this age-group is inappropriate. Individuals with a history of carditis are candidates for prophylactic treatment to prevent a recurrence of rheumatic fever, which may lead to further cardiac damage. Rest and nutrition regimens are appropriate interventions for children with rheumatic fever, but they cannot prevent recurrence of the disease. Maintaining a healthy state helps an individual to resist infection but is not an absolute safeguard against a streptococcal infection.

12 Correct answer—C

Because rheumatic fever is not an infectious disease, no particular precautions are needed to prevent its spread. Fever and anorexia increase the body's demand for calories and nutrients; therefore, adequate nutrition is a primary concern. Resting decreases the demands placed on the heart, an organ that is stressed by inflammation. Compliance with the prescribed prophylactic medication regimen is crucial. The regimen to prevent recurrence involves monthly injections of penicillin G and either two daily doses of oral penicillin or one daily dose of oral sulfadiazine. The duration of the prophylactic treatment, though uncertain, can be lengthy. The child and his family may benefit from emotional support to help them cope with the frustrating aspects of the disease, such as chorea, activity restrictions, fear of permanent heart damage, and long-term prophylactic treatment.

13 Correct answer—B

AIDS and AIDS-related complex (ARC) are diseases caused by the human immunodeficiency virus (HIV). Children with AIDS or ARC commonly have acute or chronic diarrhea. A less common manifestation of an HIV infection is microcephaly, not hydrocephaly. Pallor and vomiting are symptoms of many conditions, but they are not found in HIV-infected children.

14 Correct answer—A

An HIV-positive child should receive the same immunizations as any other child, but he should not receive live vaccines. Live viruses are not administered to any person who has an impaired immune system because of the possibility of developing a severe vaccine-induced illness. Live virus vaccines include oral polio virus (OPV) and measles, mumps, rubella (MMR). Pneumococcal vaccine is recommended only for children under age 2 with sickle cell disease, asplenia, nephrotic syndrome, or Hodgkin's disease. *Haemophilus influenzae* type B (Hib) vaccine is recommended for all children, including those with HIV, to prevent such serious childhood infections as bacterial meningitis, epiglottis, and bacterial pneumonia. It is given at ages 2, 4, 6, and 18 months. Periodic administration of immune globulin may be indicated in some HIV-infected children.

15 Correct answer—C

The day-care workers should disinfect surfaces soiled with Stephen's or Janie's blood or body fluids with a bleach solution; a solution of 1 part bleach to 10 parts water kills HIV. The workers also should wear gloves when handling body fluids or wiping contaminated surfaces. Masks are unnecessary because HIV is not transmitted by airborne particles. Barring the children from the day-care center should not be an automatic reaction. Children who are HIV-positive should be evaluated individually to determine whether they should attend day-care or school. For example, children who do not have control of body fluids or who exhibit such behaviors as biting should be excluded. HIV status should be confidential; day-care managers are not required to notify the parents of other children who attend the center.

CHAPTER 7

Emergencies

Questions

1 Most pediatric head injuries are caused by:

A. Motor vehicle accidents
B. Child abuse
C. Noncontact sports
D. Falls

2 Concussion commonly results in:

A. Persistent loss of consciousness
B. Transient loss of consciousness
C. No loss of consciousness
D. Delayed loss of consciousness

3 The temperature of a child with an injured head should:

A. Be taken orally
B. Be taken rectally
C. Be taken by the axillary route
D. Not be taken

4 Lodgment of a foreign body in a child's esophagus typically results in:

A. Coughing
B. Choking
C. Inability to speak
D. Increased salivation

5 Renal trauma commonly is associated with:

A. Hematuria
B. Fever
C. Colic
D. Polyuria

6 What is the correct hand placement for cardiac compression in an infant?

A. Above the nipple line
B. At the nipple line
C. One finger-width below the nipple line
D. At the xiphoid

7 Which is the correct ratio of breaths to compressions for infant CPR?

A. 1:5
B. 1:15
C. 2:10
D. 2:15

8 When performing cardiac compression on an infant, the nurse should compress the sternum:

A. ¼″ (0.6 cm)
B. ½″ to 1″ (1.3 to 2.5 cm)
C. 1½″ (3.8 cm)
D. 2″ (5 cm)

9 Because an infant's airways and adjuncts are small and susceptible to blockage by mucus and blood, administered oxygen should be:

A. Cooled
B. Humidified
C. At body temperature
D. Filtered

10 What is the proper way to correct air entrapment in an infant's stomach during CPR?

A. Press the abdomen
B. Insert a nasogastric tube
C. Change the ventilation method to a resuscitation bag
D. Continue ventilation but use only enough force to make the chest rise

11 The nurse selects an endotracheal tube based on the diameter of a child's:

A. Mouth
B. Cricoid cartilage
C. Glottic opening
D. Main stem bronchi

12 If the nurse is alone with a child who goes into cardiac arrest, she should immediately:

A. Administer CPR for 1 minute, then phone for help
B. Find someone to help initiate CPR
C. Shout for help once, then perform CPR until she cannot continue
D. Stay with the child and wait for help before beginning CPR

13 What is the preferred route for vascular access in a neonate?

A. Temporal vein
B. Umbilical vein
C. Femoral vein
D. Antecubital vein

14 Barbiturate poisoning is characterized by:

A. Widely dilated and reactive pupils
B. Widely dilated and fixed pupils
C. Pinpoint pupils
D. Unilaterally fixed pupils

15 Scald burns are most common among children ages:

A. 6 to 24 months
B. 2 to 4 years
C. 6 to 10 years
D. 12 to 16 years

16 Full-thickness burns cause injury to the:

A. Epidermis
B. Dermis
C. Epidermis and dermis
D. Skin and fat

SITUATION

Mrs. Todd finds her 3-year-old son, Peter, playing in the bathroom medicine chest. She discovers an open bottle of aspirin on the floor and white powder on the child's lips. She immediately calls the local emergency department (ED) for help.

Questions 17 and 18 refer to this situation.

17 Which question should the nurse ask before giving Mrs. Todd any advice over the telephone?

A. "Has the child been ill recently?"
B. "Is the child alert?"
C. "Is the child allergic to aspirin?"
D. "Has this ever happened before?"

18 The nurse correctly instructs Mrs. Todd to:

A. Give the child a glass of milk and bring him to the hospital
B. Give the child nothing to drink and bring him to the hospital immediately
C. Give the child syrup of ipecac
D. Bring the child to the hospital if she notices blood in his stool

---

SITUATION

Jeffrey, age 10, accidentally spills acid on his right leg and foot while playing with a chemistry set in his basement. He is brought to the ED by his father. Physical examination reveals second- and third-degree circumferential burns. Jeffrey weighs 55 lb (25 kg).

Questions 19 and 20 refer to this situation.

19 Which emergency treatment is most important for a burn caused by acid?

A. Rinsing the burn with a continuous stream of running water
B. Wrapping the burn with a clean sheet or towel
C. Cleaning the burn with a solution of mild soap and water
D. Wrapping the burn with sterile gauze soaked in normal saline solution

20 To decrease the potential long-term effects of Jeffrey's burns, the nurse should:

A. Maintain Jeffrey's affected foot in an extended position
B. Maintain Jeffrey's affected foot in a flexed position
C. Elevate Jeffrey's affected leg on pillows
D. Perform range-of-motion exercises on Jeffrey's affected foot and ankle

Roger, age 10, is admitted to the ED and then to the pediatric unit after being hit in the eye with a baseball. His diagnosis is traumatic hyphema. The physician prescribes bed rest and administration of timolol maleate (Timoptic) ½% and aminocaproic acid (Amicar).

Questions 21 to 24 refer to this situation.

21 The nurse's responsibilities for assessing and managing Roger in the ED include all of the following *except:*

A. Palpating the orbital rim to assess for fracture
B. Preparing for corneal staining
C. Conducting preoperative teaching and preparation
D. Irrigating the injured eye

22 The priority medical and nursing concern for Roger should be directed at:

A. Preventing rebleeding episodes
B. Preventing infection
C. Relieving anxiety
D. Relieving pain

23 Which symptom is Roger unlikely to experience?

A. Pain
B. Drowsiness
C. Nausea
D. Impaired vision in his uninjured eye

24 While Roger is receiving aminocaproic acid (Amicar), the nurse must observe for:

A. Evidence of a clotting disorder
B. Hypercalcemia
C. Fluid retention
D. Hypertension

Kelly Powers, age 6, is admitted to the ED after being involved in a motor vehicle accident. An unrestrained passenger in the front seat, she was found unconscious at the accident scene but was aroused during transport. The nurse notes that Kelly, who is now alert, has a bleeding 8-cm laceration on her front scalp.

Questions 25 to 29 refer to this situation.

25 Which nursing action is *not* a priority at this time?

A. Assessing the quality of Kelly's respirations
B. Cleaning the scalp wound
C. Administering oxygen
D. Initiating an I.V. line with a crystalloid solution

26 A scalp laceration is a significant injury in a child because:

A. A child's scalp is highly vascular and substantial blood loss is possible
B. Scarring is possible
C. The laceration places the child at high risk for infection
D. Damage to underlying nerves and blood vessels is possible

27 Bleeding from a laceration is best controlled by applying:

A. A pressure dressing
B. Direct pressure to the site
C. A tourniquet
D. Pressure to arterial pressure points

28 Which assessment finding is the most accurate indicator of altered neurologic status in a child?

A. Diminished vital signs
B. Inability to carry on a conversation
C. Decreased level of consciousness
D. Pupillary dilation

29 At discharge, the nurse should advise Kelly's parents to anticipate which complication of concussion within the next few weeks?

A. Vomiting
B. Difficulty concentrating or remembering recent events
C. Ataxia
D. Blacking out

SITUATION

Jason Coyne, age 15 months, is brought to the ED by his mother after falling down a flight of stairs. Mrs. Coyne states that she saw Jason fall down the stairs as she was putting laundry into the washer in their basement. Although Jason has no open wounds on his head, he has a rapid pulse, is hyperventilating, and is still crying.

Questions 30 to 33 refer to this situation.

30 Which question elicits the most useful baseline information from Jason's mother?

A. "When is the last time Jason ate?"
B. "Has Jason fallen down these stairs before?"
C. "Did Jason cry immediately after falling?"
D. "Did Jason's pupils seem to be of equal size when you picked him up?"

31 Which assessment finding indicates brain stem involvement?

A. Rapid pulse
B. Hyperventilation
C. Wide fluctuations in pulse rate
D. Irritability and continued crying

32 After undergoing a computed tomography (CT) scan, Jason is admitted to the hospital for a 24-hour observation period. The physician prescribes acetaminophen (Tylenol). This medication is administered to:

A. Regulate temperature
B. Control headache
C. Control seizures
D. Decrease intracranial pressure

33 When Jason is discharged, the nurse instructs his mother to call the physician immediately if Jason:

A. Cannot be aroused normally
B. Wants to sleep during the next 24 hours
C. Seems to have a headache
D. Is more irritable than usual

SITUATION

Margaret Sharp, age 3, is being treated in the ED for lead ingestion. The physician diagnoses plumbism (lead poisoning) and admits the child to the hospital. Mrs. Sharp explains to the nurse that she has three other children at home and would have difficulty finding child care and transportation to come to the hospital for appointments. She wants to know if follow-up visits are important.

Questions 34 to 38 refer to this situation.

---

34 Which intervention does *not* enhance compliance with follow-up visits?

A. Providing a thorough explanation of the treatment
B. Arranging for transportation and child care
C. Reinforcing information with written instructions
D. Using fear of long-term consequences as a motivator

---

35 Margaret's blood lead level is 80 mcg/dl and her erythrocyte-protoporphyrin level is 260 mcg/dl. Considering these findings, the nurse should inform Mrs. Sharp that:

A. The levels are within normal limits
B. Further testing is necessary
C. The levels necessitate treatment
D. Safe lead levels have yet to be established

---

36 Initial signs and symptoms of plumbism include:

A. Diarrhea, vomiting, blurred vision, and headache
B. Hyperventilation, dizziness, fever, and chills
C. Sporadic abdominal cramping, anorexia, jaundice, and confusion
D. Acute abdominal cramping, vomiting, anorexia, headache, and fever

---

37 In caring for Margaret, the nurse should be chiefly concerned with preparing the child for:

A. Blood testing
B. Receiving many injections
C. Frequent hospitalizations
D. Radiographic testing

38 Which condition is a potential untoward effect of chelation therapy?

A. Seizures
B. Diarrhea
C. Headaches
D. Muscular atrophy

Answer sheet

A B C D
1 ○○○○
2 ○○○○
3 ○○○○
4 ○○○○
5 ○○○○
6 ○○○○
7 ○○○○
8 ○○○○
9 ○○○○
10 ○○○○
11 ○○○○
12 ○○○○
13 ○○○○
14 ○○○○
15 ○○○○
16 ○○○○
17 ○○○○
18 ○○○○
19 ○○○○
20 ○○○○
21 ○○○○
22 ○○○○
23 ○○○○
24 ○○○○
25 ○○○○
26 ○○○○
27 ○○○○
28 ○○○○
29 ○○○○
30 ○○○○

A B C D
31 ○○○○
32 ○○○○
33 ○○○○
34 ○○○○
35 ○○○○
36 ○○○○
37 ○○○○
38 ○○○○

Answers and rationales

1 Correct answer—**D**

Falls are the leading cause of head injury in children of all ages; motor vehicle accidents are the second leading cause. Other common causes include violent shaking (also known as shaken baby syndrome), which is a form of abuse that typically is associated with infants and toddlers, and accidents involving bicycles and contact sports in children over age 12.

2 Correct answer—**B**

Concussion results in a transient and instantaneous loss of consciousness. The most common type of head injury, concussion is thought to occur when shearing forces are concentrated in the central brain stem. Shearing forces are caused by unequal movement or different rates of acceleration within the brain. These forces can stretch, compress, or tear nerve fibers and small arteries.

3 Correct answer—**C**

Axillary temperature assessment is the safest and least irritating method for a child with a head injury. Because a child with this type of injury is prone to irritability, vomiting, and seizures, oral and rectal temperature assessments are contraindicated. A child with an injured head initially may exhibit mild hypothermia, followed by a moderately elevated temperature for 1 to 2 days. A persistent fever may indicate subarachnoid hemorrhage or infection.

4 Correct answer—**D**

Lodgment of a foreign object in a child's esophagus typically results in increased salivation, drooling, gagging, and dysphagia. Coughing, choking, and inability to speak are associated with aspiration of an object into the respiratory tract.

5 Correct answer—**A**

The kidneys are the most commonly injured organ in children because they are more mobile and less well-protected than an adult's. Hematuria, constant flank pain, skin abrasions in the flank, and oliguria are signs and symptoms of renal trauma. Treatment may include bed rest, blood replacement, or surgery. Fever usually is not associated with renal trauma.

6 Correct answer—**C**

Before initiating cardiac compression in an infant, the nurse should visualize a line between the infant's nipples. She then should place two or three fingers on the sternum one finger-width below the imaginary line; this is the correct hand placement for performing CPR on a child under age 1. An infant's heart is positioned more horizontally than an adult's, and the apex is higher (third or fourth intercostal space versus fifth intercostal space in an older child or adult). Placing the hands above or below the designated landmark results in less effective cardiac compressions. Hand placement at the xiphoid could result in fracture and subsequent internal injuries.

7 Correct answer—**A**

To ensure adequate ventilation and circulation, the nurse should perform infant CPR at a ratio of 1:5 (one breath to five compressions). The compressions should cease during ventilation to allow for adequate lung expansion.

8 Correct answer—**B**

The infant's sternum must be compressed ½″ to 1″ (1.3 to 2.5 cm) to ensure adequate circulation during CPR. This depth sufficiently compresses the heart between the sternum and the spine to circulate blood to the vital organs. In comparison, the sternum is compressed 1″ to 1½″ (2.5 to 3.8 cm) in children and 1½″ to 2″ (3.8 to 5 cm) in adults. The nurse should keep her fingers in place during compression and relaxation to maintain correct positioning. Incorrect positioning can fracture the rib cage or xiphoid and result in internal injuries.

9 Correct answer—**B**

Humidified oxygen helps to prevent the obstruction of an airway by mucus and blood caused by loosened and liquefied secretions. Neonates have sensitive cold receptors in their facial area and immature thermoregulation abilities; therefore, oxygen should be warmed as well. Administered oxygen does not need to be filtered.

10 Correct answer—**D**

When an infant's stomach is distended with air during CPR, the nurse should continue to ventilate, using only enough force for the chest to rise. The nurse can inflate an infant's lungs sufficiently by emitting small puffs of air (breaths that are decreased in volume). Delivering large volumes of air can lead to air entrapment in the stomach. Pressing the abdomen is likely to cause regurgitation and aspiration of vomitus. Continuing ventilation is critical; inserting a nasogastric tube interferes with this procedure. A resuscitation bag may not be readily available; besides, delivering a large volume of air via the bag would contribute to, not correct, air entrapment.

11 Correct answer—B

Because a child's airway is narrowest at the cricoid cartilage, the nurse should determine which size endotracheal (ET) tube to use based on the diameter of this structure. The nurse should auscultate for bilateral breath sounds when inserting the tube and periodically suction secretions to maintain an open airway. The child's mouth and main stem bronchi have no bearing on selection of an ET tube.

12 Correct answer—A

A child (or an adult) in cardiac arrest requires immediate attention to prevent irreversible brain damage. Therefore, the nurse should begin CPR immediately. After administering CPR for 1 minute, she should phone for help and return to the child quickly.

13 Correct answer—B

The preferred route for delivering blood, fluids, and medications to a neonate is via the umbilical vein, which permits rapid access to the circulatory system. Other commonly used sites include the peripheral veins on the dorsal surface of the hands and feet and, to a lesser extent, the scalp and antecubital veins.

14 Correct answer—C

Pinpoint pupils are a sign of barbiturate or opiate poisoning. Widely dilated and reactive pupils are associated with seizures or trauma. Cranial nerve III paralysis, hypothermia, anoxia, and ischemia cause pupils to appear dilated and unreactive. Unilaterally fixed pupils are characteristic of ocular trauma, uveitis, and instillation of cycloplegic drugs.

15 Correct answer—A

Scald burns are most common in children between ages 6 and 24 months. Such burns typically result from bathing the infant in too-hot water or from spilling hot liquids. Although scald burns may be accidental, they frequently are associated with parental abuse or neglect.

16 Correct answer—C

Full-thickness burns damage the epidermis and dermis. Partial-thickness burns damage the epithelium and can extend to the corium. Superficial burns, which are extremely painful, affect only the epidermis. Burns that involve fat sometimes are known as fourth-degree burns.

17 Correct answer—B

Before instituting any emergency measures, the nurse should determine the child's level of consciousness. If the child is not alert, he may aspirate if given an emetic. The other questions do not elicit information that is pertinent to the immediate problem.

18 Correct answer—C

Because Mrs. Todd knows for certain that her son has ingested a medication and not a caustic agent, the nurse should suggest inducing vomiting with syrup of ipecac. Giving the child a glass of milk would speed absorption of the aspirin. Waiting for bleeding to occur is inappropriate, as is waiting until arrival at the hospital to begin treatment; in some instances, delayed treatment can be fatal. Salicylate ingestion can be managed at home if treatment is implemented immediately and the child has swallowed less than 300 mg/kg. If the amount ingested cannot be determined, the nurse should instruct the parent to bring the child to the hospital after giving him syrup of ipecac. At the hospital, the physician may use gastric lavage or administer activated charcoal to wash out the aspirin.

19 Correct answer—A

Acid will continue to burn as long as it is in contact with the skin. Therefore, rinsing the burn with a running stream of water is most important. After the acid has been washed away, the burn wound should be wrapped with a clean sheet or towel to prevent contamination and to minimize pain by occluding the wound. Washing with soap and water and wrapping the area with saline-soaked gauze are insufficient to dilute and neutralize the acid.

20 Correct answer—D

The long-term goal of burn treatment is to minimize loss of function. Performing range-of-motion exercises on the ankle and foot prevents joint contractures and helps to maintain optimal function. Foot drop results from maintaining the foot in an extended position. Maintaining the foot in a flexed position results in contractures from the formation of scar tissue. Elevating the leg has no effect on future function.

21 Correct answer—D

Irrigating the eye is contraindicated in this situation because the child has a buildup of blood in the eye chamber, and any additional fluid could result in increased intraocular pressure. During the initial phase of care, the nurse should assess the child's overall condition and perform or assist with any diagnostic and therapeutic procedures. During subsequent assessments, the nurse may gently palpate the orbital rim to assess for crepitus, a grinding or grating sensation detected during palpation. The cornea may be stained with fluorescein and checked under fluorescent light for corneal abrasion, a common eye injury. If the physician decides to evacuate a hematoma, the nurse must prepare the child for surgery.

22 Correct answer—A

The priority concern in traumatic hyphema is to prevent rebleeding, which can cause increased intraocular pressure and ensuing tissue damage. Although Roger may be anxious (because of the hospitalization, his decreased ability to see, or his concern over regaining his sight) or in pain from the increased intraocular pressure and trauma, relieving anxiety and pain is not the primary concern. Preventing infection also is not a priority at this time.

23 Correct answer—D

Roger should not have difficulty seeing out of his uninjured eye; if he experiences any vision loss, the nurse should report the problem to the physician immediately to investigate the cause. Roger may experience pain, drowsiness, and nausea from head trauma or increased intraocular pressure.

24 Correct answer—A

Aminocaproic acid (Amicar) inhibits fibrinolysis. It is used to enhance hemostasis in patients with hyphema and other disorders in which fibrinolysis contributes to bleeding. This medication is contraindicated in patients with active intravascular clotting. Hypercalcemia, fluid retention, and hypertension are not related to administration of aminocaproic acid.

25 Correct answer—B

Cleaning the patient's wounds is not the nurse's priority at this time; this is done after assessing and managing the child's ABCs—airway, breathing, and circulation. The nurse must ensure an adequate airway by manual positioning (such as the head-tilt, chin-lift maneuver) or insertion of an airway-management device. She should assess the child's respirations for rate, depth, and pattern and provide mouth-to-mouth or bag-valve-mask ventilation, if necessary. Because Kelly is at high risk for respiratory compromise or sudden circulatory decompensation, the nurse should administer oxygen. She also should assess the child's circulation and treat her for hypovolemic shock, if necessary. Inserting an I.V. catheter and providing fluid resuscitation also are essential.

26 Correct answer—A

A child's scalp is highly vascular, so lacerations can lead to loss of large amounts of blood. Scarring is not a significant problem on the scalp, and infection is of no greater concern in the scalp area than it is in other parts of the body. Few underlying nerves or blood vessels in the scalp are susceptible to long-term damage.

27 Correct answer—B

Direct pressure is the most effective way to control bleeding because the vessels supplying blood to the area can be manually occluded. Direct pressure can by augmented by applying pressure to the arterial pressure points, a procedure that diminishes arterial blood flow to the injury and slows bleeding. A pressure dressing does not control bleeding and can hinder wound assessment; it is used to apply pressure to the injury after the bleeding stops. A tourniquet should never be used, except in the case of an amputation, and then only with extreme caution. Incorrect use of a tourniquet not only cuts the supply of blood to the injured site but also compromises the blood supply distal to the tourniquet. Tissue ischemia and necrosis can result.

28 Correct answer—C

Decreased level of consciousness, such as lethargy or diminished response to pain, is an early indication of a child's altered neurologic status. Changes in vital signs or pupil size may not appear until significant deterioration has occurred. The ability to carry on a conversation is a poor indicator because it can be affected by other factors.

29 Correct answer—B

A head injury usually interrupts a child's cognitive processes; therefore, Kelly may have difficulty concentrating or remembering events for an indefinite period. Dizziness, double vision, irritability, and sensitivity to bright lights or loud noises also are common after a head injury. Vomiting, ataxia, or blacking out are warning signs of more serious complications, such as subdural or subarachnoid hemmorhage.

30 Correct answer—C

The nurse must first ascertain whether Jason lost consciousness. Asking about his crying provides data about his response immediately after the fall. This information can help determine the type and extent of head injury. For example, an epidural hemorrhage is marked by initial unconsciousness, followed by an asymptomatic period (up to 48 hours), then a period of lethargy. Information about eating is not pertinent. However, projectile vomiting is a sign of increased intracranial pressure and should be monitored. Whether the child has previously fallen down the stairs is not initially relevant. The nurse may want to ask this question later; recurrent injuries may be a sign of child abuse or an indication that the parents need to be taught about child safety. Pupil reaction should be checked during the neurologic assessment; the child's mother cannot be expected to remember pupil size in an emergency.

31 Correct answer—C

Although rapid pulse, hyperventilation, irritability, and pallor commonly follow a head injury, brain stem involvement is signaled by wide fluctuations in pulse or blood pressure. The brain stem controls many vital functions, including heart rate, blood pressure, and respiration. Pressure in the lower portion of the brain stem may cause bradycardia and affect arterial blood pressure. Deep, rapid, or intermittent and gasping respirations also indicate brain stem pressure. Marked hypotension may be a sign of internal injuries.

32 Correct answer—B

Acetaminophen (Tylenol) usually is administered to control headache in a patient with a head injury. Aspirin is contraindicated because it can increase bleeding, and narcotics may mask signs of increasing intracranial pressure. Although acetaminophen sometimes is used as an antipyretic, no evidence indicates that Jason's hypothalamus (temperature-regulating center) was affected by the fall. Acetaminophen does not control seizures or intracranial pressure.

33 Correct answer—A

Although the child will be sleepy from frequent neurologic checks and the stress of hospitalization, he should be able to be aroused in his normal way. His mother should allow him to sleep for some time, but she should check on him every 2 hours. Having a headache after a fall is common. Jason may be more irritable than usual because of a headache, fatigue, or disruption of his normal daily routine.

34 Correct answer—D

The nurse should review the detrimental effects of inadequate treatment but should not use fear tactics as a motivator. She should explain the significance of the disease and the need for treatment so that Mrs. Sharp will be motivated to bring her daughter to the hospital for follow-up appointments. Written materials that reinforce information are especially helpful in situations in which multiple or complex treatments are required. Lack of services, such as transportation and child care, can pose an obstacle to parents; arranging for these services may increase the mother's compliance with the follow-up schedule.

35 Correct answer—C

Plumbism is defined as two successive blood lead levels of 70 mcg/dl or more, or a blood lead level of 50 mcg/dl and an erythrocyte-protoprophyrin level of 250 mcg/dl or more. Symptoms may or may not be present. Children who are diagnosed with lead poisoning on the basis of these levels require treatment. Chelation therapy is used to rid the body of lead by combining it with another substance.

36 Correct answer—D

The initial signs and symptoms of plumbism include headache, fever, vomiting, acute abdominal cramping, and anorexia. Long-term effects include anemia, glycosuria, proteinuria, ketonuria, behavioral changes, mental retardation, paralysis, blindness, coma, and death. Lead encephalopathy can cause slight behavioral changes, such as hyperactivity, lethargy, irritability, learning difficulties, and short attention span. As the lead levels increase, the child's intellectual capacity decreases.

37 Correct answer—B

Because chelation therapy involves numerous injections, the nurse should prepare Margaret for receiving injections by means of role playing and age-appropriate explanations. Disodium calcium and dimercaprol are administered as separate injections; these viscous solutions cause discomfort. The nurse should encourage Margaret to express her pain and assure her, in age-appropriate terms, that the therapy is not punishment for eating lead or paint. Treatment for lead poisoning does not require frequent hospitalizations; however, frequent outpatient follow-up is crucial. Radiographic and blood testing play a role in diagnosis; they provide information about the amount of lead in a child's body. After diagnosis, they are used less frequently. These procedures are less painful and less traumatic than chelation therapy.

38 Correct answer—A

Initially, chelation therapy can cause severe and possibly fatal seizures from the rapid rise of serum lead levels. Chelation mobilizes the lead from soft tissue and bone, then combines the lead with a stable substance that is excreted through the kidneys. Chelating agents enhance urinary excretion 20- to 50-fold. Diarrhea, headaches, and muscular atrophy are unrelated to this therapy.

CHAPTER 8

Elimination

Questions

1 A neonate has a decreased ability to resorb:

A. Potassium
B. Sodium
C. Urea
D. Hydrogen

2 Signs and symptoms of urinary tract infection in a child ages 1 to 2 typically include:

A. Poor feeding and vomiting
B. Rash and edema
C. Fatigue and irritability
D. Restlessness and tremor

3 Nephrotic syndrome results from:

A. Glomerular injury
B. Ureteral injury
C. Bladder trauma
D. Meatal constriction

4 The nurse's primary responsibility in caring for a child with nephrotic syndrome is to:

A. Provide opportunities for increased physical activity
B. Provide frequent repositioning and turning
C. Encourage a high-sodium diet
D. Encourage fluid intake

5 Acute renal failure in children most commonly is caused by:

A. Dehydration
B. Hypertension
C. Renal infection
D. Cancer

6 One of the nurse's primary responsibilities when caring for a child with acute renal failure is to:

A. Measure fluid status
B. Lower the environmental temperature
C. Provide opportunities for physical activity
D. Encourage a high-protein diet

7 James, age 2, is admitted to the hospital for surgical repair of hypospadias. Postoperatively, the child should be maintained in which position?

A. High-Fowler's
B. Supine
C. Prone
D. Semi-Fowler's

8 Which side effect is most common after hemodialysis?

A. Seizures
B. Irritability
C. Restlessness
D. Tremor

9 A neonate typically passes meconium stool within how many hours after delivery?

A. 4 to 6
B. 6 to 10
C. 10 to 24
D. 24 to 36

10 Constipation is most common in children ages:

A. 6 to 12 months
B. 12 to 18 months
C. 1 to 3 years
D. 3 to 5 years

11 What is the most common reason for abdominal surgery in a child over age 2?

A. Appendicitis
B. Phimosis
C. Inguinal hernia
D. Hydrocele

12 Appendicitis is associated with colicky abdominal pain, tenderness, and:

  A. Fever
  B. Pallor
  C. Restlessness
  D. Fatigue

13 Postoperative nursing care after an appendectomy for a ruptured appendix includes:

  A. Maintaining the patient in a semi-Fowler's position
  B. Positioning the patient on the left side
  C. Auscultating bowel sounds every other day
  D. Caring for the patient's colostomy

14 Which statement about ulcerative colitis is *true?*

  A. It is rare in children
  B. It affects adults only
  C. It typically develops at about age 11
  D. It affects adolescents only

15 A child with ulcerative colitis should follow which type of diet?

  A. Low protein
  B. High protein
  C. Low calorie
  D. High fat

16 Crohn's disease commonly manifests as anorexia, lethargy, fatigue, and:

  A. Fever
  B. Cyanosis
  C. Constipation
  D. Acute abdominal pain

17 Which type of hepatitis is transmitted by the oral-fecal route?

  A. Hepatitis A
  B. Hepatitis B
  C. Hepatitis P
  D. Hepatitis C (non-A, non-B)

SITUATION

Jacki, age 4, is brought to the pediatrician's office after experiencing nonprojectile, nonbilious vomiting, fever, and coffee-colored urine for the past day. Her history reveals that she was well until 2 weeks ago, when she developed a sore throat that was uncultured and untreated. Her vital signs are: temperature, 102° F (38.9° C); blood pressure, 134/76 mm Hg; pulse rate, 76 beats/minute; and respiratory rate, 24 breaths/minute. Urinalysis shows hematuria and proteinuria. Jacki is admitted to the hospital for evaluation. Laboratory analyses reveal a positive antistreptolysin titer, elevated blood urea nitrogen (BUN) and creatinine levels, and decreased creatinine clearance. The physician diagnoses acute glomerulonephritis (AGN).

Questions 18 to 23 refer to this situation.

---

18 Which organism is commonly responsible for AGN?

A. Group A beta-hemolytic streptococci
B. *Staphylococcus epidermis*
C. *Pseudomonas aeruginosa*
D. *Escherichia coli*

---

19 An increased BUN level and a decreased creatinine clearance usually indicate:

A. Metabolic alkalosis
B. Glomerular damage
C. Liver damage
D. Bladder damage

---

20 The nurse would expect Jacki to exhibit which assessment finding on admission?

A. Puffiness in the periorbital area
B. Circumoral pallor
C. High fever and positive throat culture for streptococci
D. Weight loss and abdominal distention

---

21 Nursing interventions for Jacki should include:

A. Encouraging her to eat high-sodium, high-protein foods
B. Administering antibiotics
C. Administering antihypertensive drugs
D. Encouraging her to eat high-potassium foods

22 Jacki complains of headaches and dizziness, and her blood pressure remains elevated. These signs and symptoms most likely indicate the development of:

A. Acute renal failure
B. Cardiac decompensation
C. Pulmonary edema
D. Encephalopathy

23 Which intervention should the nurse include in the care plan of a child with AGN who has cardiac decompensation?

A. Assessing urine specific gravity hourly
B. Encouraging ambulation
C. Monitoring daily weight
D. Encouraging fluid intake

SITUATION

Stuart, a normally healthy 8-month-old infant, is admitted to the hospital for gastroenteritis. The nurse notices that he is irritable, has a depressed anterior fontanel, and has severe diarrhea. His vital signs are: blood pressure, 70/30 mm Hg; pulse rate, 110 beats/minute; respiratory rate, 50 breaths/minute; and temperature, 104° F (40° C) rectally.

Questions 24 to 26 refer to this situation.

24 Gastroenteritis is best described as:

A. An inflammation in the wall of the stomach
B. An inflammation in the stomach and intestines
C. An infectious disease in the abdomen caused by bacteria
D. A disease of unknown etiology that causes diarrhea and emesis

25 Which nursing action is *not* appropriate during Stuart's initial stabilization?

A. Administering an antidiarrheal medication
B. Monitoring his intake and output closely
C. Withholding his formula
D. Recording his stool history

26 If Stuart's gastroenteritis were to continue without treatment, he probably will develop:

A. Metabolic alkalosis
B. Metabolic acidosis
C. Respiratory alkalosis
D. Respiratory acidosis

SITUATION

Linda, age 10 months, is sent to the pediatric unit of the hospital directly from her pediatrician's office. She has had large, watery green stools for the past 24 hours, and she cannot retain formula. She has lost about $3^1/_2$ lb (1.5 kg) since her last pediatric visit. She is mottled, lethargic, and dehydrated. Her extremities are clammy, and peripheral pulses are decreased. Arterial blood gas (ABG) analysis reveals pH, 7.2; $Paco_2$, 22 mm Hg; Pao_2, 96 mm Hg; HCO_3^-, 22 mEq/liter; and base excess, −18.

Questions 27 to 29 refer to this situation.

---

27 Which acid-base disorder does Linda have?

A. Metabolic alkalosis
B. Metabolic acidosis
C. Respiratory alkalosis
D. Respiratory acidosis

---

28 The nurse's highest priority in caring for Linda is to:

A. Initiate reverse isolation
B. Monitor Linda's intake, output, and hydration status
C. Administer antibiotics
D. Administer adsorbants, such as kaolin and pectin

---

29 Dehydration is a common complication of severe diarrhea in infants. Which sign indicates severe dehydration?

A. Pallor
B. Decreased blood pressure
C. Polyuria
D. Bulging fontanels

SITUATION

Philip, age 10 months, is brought to the emergency department by his parents, who report that he has experienced nonprojectile, nonbilious vomiting off and on for 1 day. He cries and pulls his legs up to his abdomen, then appears normal for awhile. He strains to have a bowel movement, which results in the passage of a bloodtinged, jelly-like stool. Physical examination reveals that Philip is irritable and crying, with decreased bowel sounds and abdominal distention. He has poor skin turgor, dry mucous membranes, and no tears. He is admitted to the hospital for a laboratory workup.

On admission, Philip's vital signs are: temperature, 100.2° F (37.9° C); blood pressure, 90/60 mm Hg; and pulse rate, 110 beats/minute; his respiratory rate is impossible to gauge because of his constant crying. The physician orders a barium enema, which reveals ileocecal intussusception, then advises the nurse to prepare Philip for surgery.

Questions 30 to 32 refer to this situation.

30 Which sign is the most reliable indicator of intussusception?

A. Constipation
B. Currant jelly stools
C. Distended abdomen
D. Diarrhea

31 The nurse ensures that Philip has adequate kidney function before adding potassium to his I.V. fluids. She does this because hyperkalemia can lead to:

A. Hemodilution
B. Fatigue
C. Cardiac arrest
D. Hepatic failure

32 Philip has a nasogastric (NG) tube in place after surgery. Which finding indicates that the tube should *not* be removed?

A. Passage of flatus
B. Passage of a normal stool
C. Return of bowel sounds
D. Decreased amount of drainage from the NG tube

SITUATION

Brian Ward, age 2, is diagnosed with Hirschsprung's disease after undergoing a series of X-rays and examination by a pediatric gastrointestinal specialist. He is admitted to the hospital for surgery. According to Mrs. Ward, Brian has chronic constipation, strange stools, and a big belly. He is much smaller than his twin brother. Brian has been on stool softeners and a low-residue diet for several months with no success.

Questions 33 to 40 refer to this situation.

33 Brian is scheduled for a bowel biopsy. Which of the following is absent in Hirschsprung's disease?

A. Intestinal fibers
B. Bile
C. Ganglion cells
D. Elastic fibers

34 The stools of a child with Hirschsprung's disease are best described as:

A. Bulky and poorly formed
B. Currant jelly-like
C. Ribbon- or pellet-like
D. Fatty and foul-smelling

35 On Brian's first day of admission, the physician prescribes a clear liquid diet. Which food is permitted with this type of diet?

A. Whole milk
B. Orange juice
C. Kool-Aid
D. Chicken noodle soup

36 The nurse must administer enemas to clear Brian's bowel of stool before surgery. Which type of enema is appropriate?

A. Soap suds solution
B. Isotonic saline solution
C. Tap water
D. Hypertonic phosphate solution

37 Brian has a colostomy, an NG tube, an I.V. line, and an indwelling urinary catheter in place after surgery. On the second postoperative day, the nurse notes that Brian's abdomen is distended. She should:

A. Check the patency of the NG tube
B. Check for bowel sounds
C. Check the suture line
D. Administer a pain medication

38 Mrs. Ward tells the nurse that Brian is in pain. Which symptom indicates that Brian is in pain?

A. Tense body position
B. Restlessness
C. Inability to be comforted
D. All of the above

39 How long should the nurse listen while auscultating Brian's bowel sounds?

A. 30 seconds
B. 2 to 5 minutes
C. 10 minutes
D. Until she hears them

40 The nurse formulates a nursing diagnosis of *Knowledge deficit related to ostomy care.* Which goal is most appropriate for Brian's parents?

A. Mr. and Mrs. Ward will demonstrate emptying and application of the ostomy appliance before Brian's discharge
B. Mr. and Mrs. Ward will describe the procedure for changing the ostomy appliance
C. The nurse will apply an occlusive ointment around the stoma
D. The nurse will teach Mr. and Mrs. Ward to observe for skin excoriation

Answer sheet

	A	B	C	D			A	B	C	D
1	○	○	○	○		31	○	○	○	○
2	○	○	○	○		32	○	○	○	○
3	○	○	○	○		33	○	○	○	○
4	○	○	○	○		34	○	○	○	○
5	○	○	○	○		35	○	○	○	○
6	○	○	○	○		36	○	○	○	○
7	○	○	○	○		37	○	○	○	○
8	○	○	○	○		38	○	○	○	○
9	○	○	○	○		39	○	○	○	○
10	○	○	○	○		40	○	○	○	○
11	○	○	○	○						
12	○	○	○	○						
13	○	○	○	○						
14	○	○	○	○						
15	○	○	○	○						
16	○	○	○	○						
17	○	○	○	○						
18	○	○	○	○						
19	○	○	○	○						
20	○	○	○	○						
21	○	○	○	○						
22	○	○	○	○						
23	○	○	○	○						
24	○	○	○	○						
25	○	○	○	○						
26	○	○	○	○						
27	○	○	○	○						
28	○	○	○	○						
29	○	○	○	○						
30	○	○	○	○						

Answers and rationales

1 Correct answer—**B**

A neonate has a reduced ability to resorb sodium and water. An infant's urine is dilute, and hydrogen ion excretion is reduced until age 1. These differences in renal function make a neonate susceptible to acidosis.

2 Correct answer—**A**

A urinary tract infection in a child ages 1 to 2 typically manifests as poor feeding, vomiting, failure to gain weight, thirst, fever, and pallor. The child also may strain or scream when urinating. A child ages 2 to 14 may develop enuresis, incontinence, and frequent urination in response to an infection.

3 Correct answer—**A**

Nephrotic syndrome, which results from glomerular injury, is characterized by gross proteinuria, edema, hypoalbuminia, and hyperlipidemia. Normally, the membrane of the glomerulus is impermeable to proteins and other large molecules. In nephrotic syndrome, the membrane loses its permeability, enabling proteins to filter into in the urine. This results in a fluid shift that is manifested clinically by edema. Idiopathic causes or exposure to drugs, heavy metals, venom, or stings can produce this disorder. Nephrotic syndrome sometimes follows acute or chronic glomerulonephritis, collagen disease, sickle cell disease, or cancer. It is not related to ureteral injury or meatal constriction.

4 Correct answer—**B**

A child in the edematous phase of the nephrotic syndrome typically is placed on bed rest and consequently is at increased risk for skin breakdown from massive edema. Because edema can limit movement, the nurse must continually turn and reposition the child to prevent tissue damage. She must pay special attention to the legs, sacrum, abdomen, and scrotum—areas that are highly susceptible to breakdown and infection. A child with nephrotic syndrome typically receives a fluid- and sodium-restricted diet; strict monitoring of intake and output is essential. Although initially lethargic, the child will need some physical activity when the edema decreases.

5 Correct answer—**A**

Acute renal failure is a sudden inability of the kidneys to regulate the volume and composition of urine in relation to the body's needs. In children, acute renal failure is a transitory condition that commonly results from dehydration or hypovolemia. Burns, hemorrhage, trauma, cardiac disease, and shock can cause the decreased kidney perfusion that results in acute renal failure.

6 Correct answer—**A**

A child with acute renal failure is at risk for fluid and electrolyte imbalances because of the kidneys' inability to respond appropriately to changing body needs. Therefore, the nurse must carefully monitor the child's fluid status. Specific nursing measures include monitoring daily weight, measuring intake and output, monitoring vital signs, measuring urine specific gravity, and observing for signs of dehydration and fluid overload. The environmental temperature should remain neutral (normal room temperature) to minimize tissue catabolism. A child with renal failure is acutely ill and has a diminished activity tolerance. Because the child typically receives only I.V. fluids, diet is not a concern. However, if the child can tolerate oral feedings, the nurse should provide low-protein foods.

7 Correct answer—**B**

Hypospadias is a congenital condition in which the opening of the urethral meatus is located on the undersurface of the penis. A child who has had surgery to repair this defect should be placed in a supine position to avoid pressure on the genitals and the incision. Placing the child in a high-Fowler's, semi-Fowler's, or prone position puts too much stress on the surgical site and may cause discomfort or disturb the incision.

8 Correct answer—**A**

Seizures commonly occur during or after hemodialysis. Although the exact cause of such seizures is unknown, researchers think that cerebral edema and hyponatremia may contribute to onset. Because seizures are most likely to occur when hemodialysis is first started, the nurse should monitor the child closely at this time. She should implement safety measures (seizure precautions) to prevent injury should a seizure occur. Emergency equipment also should be readily available. Irritability, restlessness, and tremor are not associated with hemodialysis.

9 Correct answer—**D**

Meconium consists of digestive tract secretions (mucus and bile), cast-off epithelial cells, and residue from swallowing amniotic fluid. The tarry green-black meconium stool is passed during the first 24 to 36 hours after birth. If meconium is not passed within 36 hours, intestinal atresia or stenosis or a congenital aganglionic or meconium plug should be suspected.

10 Correct answer—**C**

Children between ages 1 and 3 are most likely to experience constipation because of environmental and dietary changes—for example, traveling or not eating enough fruits and vegetables. Placing the child on a high-fiber diet generally helps. If constipation persists, a stool softener, such as docusate sodium (Colace), may be needed.

11 Correct answer—**A**

Appendicitis (inflammation of the appendix)—the most common cause of pediatric abdominal surgery—can occur in all age-groups, but it rarely occurs in children under age 2. Untreated appendicitis can result in peritonitis. Phimosis is a narrowing of the foreskin opening; surgical repair (indicated only in severe cases) involves circumcision, which is not considered abdominal surgery. Inguinal hernia repair is the most common surgical procedure in infants. Hydrocele—a circumscribed collection of fluid typically found in the testicle or along the spermatic cord— usually resolves spontaneously; surgery is not required unless the hydrocele persists beyond age 1.

12 Correct answer—**A**

Colicky abdominal pain, tenderness, and a low-grade fever are the most common signs and symptoms of appendicitis.

13 Correct answer—**A**

Maintaining the patient in a semi-Fowler's position or placing him on his right side promotes drainage from the peritoneal cavity and decreases abscess formation. Placing the child on his right side also helps to confine the infection to the right lower quadrant;

placing him on his left side is contraindicated because abdominal fluid could flow into the left lower quadrant, thereby spreading the infection. The nurse must auscultate bowel sounds frequently (at least once per shift). The presence of bowel sounds indicates the return of peristalsis. A colostomy is not performed for appendicitis.

14 Correct answer—C

Ulcerative colitis—a chronic inflammatory bowel disease involving the mucosa and submucosa of the large intestine—typically develops at about age 11. Although the etiology of this disorder is unclear, genetic and environmental influences may play a role in its development. In children with this disease, the mucus membrane of the large intestine becomes hyperemic and edematous, which leads to bleeding and ulceration. The injured intestinal mucosa interferes with resorption of fluid, electrolytes, and food substances, resulting in diarrhea and growth retardation.

15 Correct answer—B

A child with ulcerative colitis loses protein from the ulcerated bowel and through bleeding. He also loses calories through the gastrointestinal tract because of impaired absorption by the affected bowel. Because ulcerative colitis is associated with a high incidence of anorexia, the child typically suffers additional protein and calorie losses. Thus, a pediatric patient with ulcerative colitis should follow a diet that is high in protein and calories and low in fat and fiber. A low-fat, low-fiber diet minimizes bowel irritation.

16 Correct answer—A

Crohn's disease is a chronic inflammatory bowel disease characterized by edema, inflammation, and ulceration of the terminal ileum. All layers of the bowel wall are affected, and the lesions are distributed in a patchy pattern with areas of healthy bowel interspersed. This pattern is different from that of ulcerative colitis, in which the lesions are contiguous. As with ulcerative colitis, the etiology of Crohn's disease is unknown, but it may be influenced by genetic and environmental factors. In the pediatric population, Crohn's disease is most common in adolescents. It manifests as anorexia, lethargy, fever, fatigue, cramping, abdominal pain and aching, diarrhea, weight loss, pallor, and anemia. These signs and symptoms are related to bowel inflammation, blood loss through the gastrointestinal tract, and the inability of the affected bowel to absorb nutrients.

17 Correct answer—**A**

Previously known as infectious hepatitis, hepatitis A is transmitted primarily by the oral-fecal route. This highly contagious disease usually is acquired through ingesting contaminated food and water. In children, hepatitis A is seen predominately in those under age 15 who live in crowded housing conditions. Children who attend day-care centers also may be exposed to the virus (transmission typically occurs through day-care workers who come in contact with contaminated diapers). Children with hepatitis A may be asymptomatic or have mild symptoms, such as nausea and vomiting, anorexia, malaise, fatigue, and fever. Jaundice may appear 5 to 7 days after infection and last up to 4 weeks. Hepatitis B is transmitted via the parenteral route. Hepatitis C (non-A, non-B) commonly is transmitted via blood transfusions. Hepatitis P does not exist.

18 Correct answer—**A**

Acute glomerulonephritis (AGN) typically occurs 10 to 14 days after infection with a nephrotogenic strain of group A beta-hemolytic streptococci. An antigen-antibody reaction to the streptococcal infection forms immune complexes that become trapped in the glomerulus. Injury and inflammation result, and the membrane becomes more porous. The patient typically is anorexic and may complain of pain; any weight gain is caused by edema.

19 Correct answer—**B**

Blood urea nitrogen (BUN) and creatinine levels are affected by kidney function and reflect glomerular filtration. An increased BUN level and a decreased creatinine clearance are signs of a decreased glomerular filtration rate, indicating glomerular damage. Metabolic alkalosis is evident in serum pH levels. BUN and creatinine levels do not reflect liver function, nor do they indicate bladder damage.

20 Correct answer—**A**

When a patient's glomerular filtration rate decreases, the body retains sodium and water, resulting in hypervolemia. Fluid retention also may contribute to hypertension, generalized edema, and weight gain; puffiness around the eyes is an initial sign of this condition. Circumoral pallor, high fever, and abdominal distention are not associated with AGN. Throat cultures for streptococci are seldom positive.

21 Correct answer—C

Antihypertensive drugs are used to control blood pressure, which is elevated in patients with AGN because of fluid and sodium retention. Although a low-sodium diet is helpful in treating hypertension, the benefit of a high- or low-protein diet is controversial. Antibiotics usually are administered only when streptococcal infection persisits; they do not affect the course of the disease. The child should avoid eating high-potassium foods because increased potassium blood levels may trigger arrhythmias.

22 Correct answer—D

Hypertensive encephalopathy is a serious complication that may develop during the acute stage of AGN. Normally, blood vessels constrict in response to acute arterial hypertension. In acute and severe hypertension, this protective response can fail, resulting in hyperfusion of the brain, cerebral edema, and increased intracranial pressure. Hypertensive encephalopathy initially manifests as headache, dizziness, vomiting, and lethargy. Although acute renal failure, cardiac decompensation, and pulmonary edema are potential complications of AGN, the symptoms reported by Jacki are not associated with these disorders.

23 Correct answer—C

The nurse must monitor the fluid balance of a child with AGN and cardiac decompensation because any fluid overload would tax the child's cardiac system and exacerbate the kidneys. Monitoring the child's daily weight is the best way to assess for fluid balance. The child should be weighed on the same scale before breakfast, wearing similar clothing each day. If the child has a restricted fluid intake and has lost a significant amount of weight, the nurse should assess for dehydration. In the acute phase of AGN, urine specific gravity usually is elevated because of altered renal function; therefore, it would not be a reliable indicator of fluid status. Ambulation would stress the child's already compromised cardiac function. Because cardiac decompensation in AGN is related to hypervolemia, oral fluid intake usually is restricted.

24 Correct answer—**B**

Gastroenteritis, an inflammation of the stomach and intestines, usually is caused by a virus, although it also may be caused by bacterial infection. Gastroenteritis is a leading cause of pediatric illness (second only to respiratory tract infections) that affects all age-groups. The severity of symptoms depends on the causative organism and may include diarrhea, vomiting, abdominal discomfort, and possibly fever.

25 Correct answer—**A**

Antidiarrheals are contraindicated in acute gastroenteritis. In most cases, diarrhea is better left untreated in a child. Antidiarrheal medications inhibit peristalsis, causing fluid retention in the bowel. This can exacerbate dehydration and electrolyte imbalance. Monitoring intake and output is essential because the child can quickly become dehydrated and develop acid-base imbalances. Dehydration that produces circulatory compromise can lead to shock. Because specific stool characteristics are associated with certain disorders, the child's stool history (consistency, frequency, color, and amount) may help identify the cause of gastroenteritis. Also, the frequency and amount of stool provides important information about fluid loss. Many children with gastroenteritis develop a secondary lactase deficiency, resulting in a temporary intolerance to milk and exacerbation of diarrhea. Therefore, milk products are withheld initially in these patients.

26 Correct answer—**B**

Metabolic acidosis associated with severe gastroenteritis can result from the cumulative effect of the loss of sodium, potassium, and bicarbonate in the intestinal tract; decreased urine output and retention of metabolites and hydrogen ions; increased lactic acid caused by tissue hypoxia; or ketosis resulting from reduced glycogen stores and fat metabolism.

27 Correct answer—**B**

Metabolic acidosis is caused by dehydration; in this case, it may be the result of loss of bicarbonate ions through diarrhea. Partial respiratory compensation for the metabolic acidosis is seen in the child's low $Paco_2$ level. A low bicarbonate ion concentration confirms that the acidosis is metabolic in origin.

28 Correct answer—B

The nurse must carefully assess the hydration of an infant with severe diarrhea. This includes accurately measuring the volume and frequency of urination, diarrhea, and vomiting, as well as the amount of fluid the infant receives per hour. The infant should be placed on enteric precautions, not reverse isolation, to prevent the spread of diarrhea. Enteric precautions include handling and disposal of enteric matter (vomitus and stool) according to hospital guidelines. Typically, the child is placed in an isolation room, and hospital personnel wear gloves and gowns when providing care. Antibiotics may or may not be necessary; such measures are initiated after the effects of dehydration are controlled. Adsorbents decrease the frequency of evacuation but do not reduce fluid loss.

29 Correct answer—B

Severe dehydration in an infant is defined as a loss of more than 15% of total body weight. A dehydrated infant typically exhibits decreased blood pressure, cyanosis or mottling, oliguria or azotemia, sunken eyeballs, depressed or sunken fontanels, dry mucous membranes, poor skin turgor, decreased tear production, pronounced tachycardia, and shocklike symptoms.

30 Correct answer—B

Intussusception is the invagination or telescoping of a portion of the bowel into an adjoining part, resulting in an obstruction. The classic signs of intussusception are vomiting, intermittent abdominal pain, and currant jelly stools (stools that take on the appearance of red currant jelly because of the large amount of blood and mucus in them).

31 Correct answer—C

Hyperkalemia can lead to the development of ventricular arrhythmias, including ventricular fibrillation and cardiac arrest. A child with decreased kidney function, increased potassium intake, accelerated tissue catabolism, or acidosis is at increased risk for hyperkalemia.

32 Correct answer—D

A reduced amount of drainage from a nasogastric (NG) tube may indicate that the tube is blocked. The passage of flatus or a normal stool and the return of bowel sounds signal that bowel function is returning and the NG tube may be discontinued.

33 Correct answer—C

A patient with Hirschsprung's disease has no parasympathetic ganglion cells in the affected portion of the colon. Because ganglion cells affect peristaltic wave transmission, their absence leads to decreased motility of bowel contents and bowel obstruction. Signs of Hirschsprung's disease in neonates include failure to pass meconium within 48 hours, poor fluid intake, bile-stained vomitus, and abdominal distention. Infants with this disease may exhibit failure to thrive, constipation, abdominal distention, and episodes of vomiting and diarrhea. In older children, Hirschsprung's disease manifests as constipation, abdominal distention, and visible peristalsis. Surgery is the primary treatment.

34 Correct answer—C

Ribbon- or pellet-like stools are characteristic of a child with Hirschsprung's disease. Currant jelly-like stools are characteristic of a child with intussusception. Bulky, poorly formed stools that are fatty and foul-smelling are associated with celiac disease.

35 Correct answer—C

Kool-Aid is the only clear (transparent) liquid listed.

36 Correct answer—B

An isotonic saline solution prevents fluid imbalances. Soap suds or hypertonic phosphate solutions can lead to diarrhea and hyperphosphatemia. Tap water is inappropriate because it can cause a fluid shift.

37 Correct answer—A

An NG tube is inserted postoperatively to promote gastric decompression, or escape of air from the stomach. A plugged tube causes the abdomen to distend rapidly from the buildup of trapped air in the stomach and intestines. Because air is trapped in the gastrointestinal tract from lack of peristalsis, bowel sounds would be absent. Checking the suture line is unnecessary. No evidence indicates that Brian is in pain.

38 Correct answer—D

Toddlers generally react to pain by displaying vigorous physical resistance and emotional upset. Persistent discomfort may result in whimpering, crying, a tense body posture, irritability, poor appetite, resistance to being left alone, and an inability to be comforted.

39 Correct answer—B

The nurse should auscultate bowel sounds in each of the child's four abdominal quadrants. When assessing these sounds, she should listen for 2 to 5 minutes. Bowel sounds typically occur every 10 to 30 seconds, depending on the bowel's activity. To determine whether bowel sounds are absent, the nurse should auscultate for at least 5 minutes.

40 Correct answer—A

Demonstration of emptying and applying the ostomy appliance is the most appropriate goal for Brian's parents; the knowledge that the nurse is attempting to impart is best taught by demonstration. Although parents may be able to describe the procedure, they may not necessarily know how to perform it correctly. Applying an occlusive ointment around the stoma does not foster parental knowledge about ostomy care. Teaching the parents about skin excoriation is not an appropriate goal. Goals should be focused on the patient's needs and accomplishments, not the nurse's.

CHAPTER 9

Cancer

Questions

SITUATION

Jerome Klein, age 6, has had a fever ranging from 99.7° to 102.2° F (37.6° to 39° C) for the past 4 days. He also has a runny nose, cough, and generalized aches and pains in his bones. His pediatrician observes pallor, ecchymoses on his legs, and petechiae on his neck and chest. Jerome also has splenomegaly; several enlarged, firm submandibular lymph nodes; and a reddened throat. The pediatrician orders a complete blood count (CBC), a platelet count, a differential, and a monospot test. The results are: white blood cell count, 600,000/mm³; hemoglobin, 7 g/dl; hematocrit, 21%; platelet count, 22,000/mm³; neutrophils, 5%; lymphocytes, 7%; lymphoblasts, 88%; and monospot test, negative.

Jerome is admitted to the hospital, where the pediatric hematologist-oncologist performs a bone marrow aspiration. He confirms the pediatrician's diagnosis of acute lymphoblastic leukemia (ALL).

Questions 1 to 5 refer to this situation.

1 The nurse's priority in treating a child with newly diagnosed ALL is to:

A. Decrease the risk of infection
B. Decrease environmental overstimulation
C. Ensure proper nutrition
D. Determine the child's concept of death

2 Based on Jerome's CBC results, neutropenic and thrombocytopenic precautions are indicated. Which of the following is *not* one of the nurse's responsibilities?

A. Limiting the number of venipunctures Jerome receives
B. Avoiding taking Jerome's temperature rectally
C. Instructing Jerome's parents on the need to limit his activities
D. Giving glycerin suppositories to decrease straining at defecation

3 Jerome begins his chemotherapeutic regimen, which consists of vincristine (Oncovin), asparaginase (Elspar), doxorubicin (Adriamycin), and prednisone (Orasone). Which nursing intervention is *not* necessary for a patient receiving prednisone?

A. Monitoring sodium intake
B. Encouraging food intake
C. Obtaining daily weights
D. Monitoring blood pressure

4 Besides his chemotherapeutic regimen, Jerome receives allopurinol (Zyloprim). The reason for this action is that allopurinol:

A. Acidifies the urine to prevent uric acid formation
B. Prevents hyperuricemic nephropathy
C. Acts synergistically with the chemotherapeutic agents to produce tumor lysis
D. Prevents kidney tissue damage, a side effect of doxorubicin

5 Extensive parent teaching is required before Jerome is discharged from the hospital. The nurse realizes that:

A. It is best to withhold some information initially and teach in short sessions after discharge
B. It is best to review all information once and then answer questions as they arise
C. It is best to provide a basic level of teaching to families under stress; information may need to be repeated many times
D. It is best to use patient-parent information booklets to teach the family about leukemia and related issues

SITUATION

Bill, age 17, was diagnosed with ALL at age 2. His induction therapy consisted of vincristine, prednisone, asparaginase, and intrathecal methotrexate. Consolidation, or intensification, therapy consisted of spinal taps with intrathecal methotrexate and cranial irradiation. Maintenance therapy involved administration of 6-mercaptopurine, methotrexate, vincristine, prednisone, and intrathecal methotrexate. Therapy was discontinued 3 years after diagnosis because Bill remained in complete, continuous remission.

Questions 6 to 8 refer to this situation.

6 When plotting a growth curve, the nurse practitioner notices that Bill was in the 50th percentile for height and weight when he was receiving chemotherapy. Since then, his height has fallen to the fifth percentile and his weight has fallen to the tenth percentile. A workup to determine the reason for this decreased growth should include all of the following *except:*

A. Endocrinologic consultation
B. Thyroid function studies
C. Wrist X-rays
D. Growth hormone injections

7 The nurse practitioner recognizes that many adolescents and young adults are long-term survivors of childhood cancer. As recently as 1970, there were very few survivors. Which factor has contributed to a change in childhood cancer survival rate?

A. Use of the three modalities of treatment—surgery, radiation, and chemotherapy
B. Use of adjuvant and combination chemotherapy
C. Use of clinical trials (treatment of patients according to investigational protocols) to continually improve survival statistics
D. All of the above

8 Bill asks why he must continue to come for follow-up checkups when he has had no problems, no medication, and no cancer for 12 years. The nurse practitioner correctly states:

A. "We must keep your records up to date"
B. "We are looking for side effects of your treatment"
C. "We need to monitor for signs of continued immuno-suppression"
D. "We need to monitor for the latent effects of your treatment and disease"

SITUATION

Danielle, age 16, was diagnosed 2 weeks ago with Hodgkin's disease stage IIIB. This diagnosis was determined by cervical node biopsy and radiographic studies.

Questions 9 to 11 refer to this situation.

9 Danielle's disease is classified as stage B rather than stage A because of the manifestation of which symptoms?

A. Hepatomegaly, splenomegaly, and fever
B. Weight loss, fever, and night sweats
C. Anorexia, malaise, and lassitude
D. Pruritus, lymphadenopathy greater than 5 cm, and splenomegaly

10 Because Danielle's chemotherapy will involve the administration of eight drugs, the nurse suggests the insertion of a venous access device. In choosing the type of device to be used, the nurse must consider:

A. The size of the veins
B. The size of the child
C. The expected use
D. The surgeon's preference

11 Danielle's medication protocols include ABVD (Adriamycin, bleomycin, vinblastine, and dacarbazine) and MOPP (nitrogen mustard, vincristine [Oncovin], prednisone, and procarbazine). To increase compliance, the nurse recommends all of the following *except:*

A. Taking the oral medications at mealtimes
B. Taking the oral medications during after-school activities
C. Pairing the medication regimens with hygiene regimens
D. Self-monitoring for side effects

SITUATION

Lori Sowenski, age 12, is admitted to the hospital complaining of headaches, early morning vomiting, and paresthesia; these symptoms have persisted for the past 2 months. A workup reveals that Lori has medulloblastoma. She undergoes surgery to debulk the tumor, and a shunt is inserted to relieve cerebrospinal fluid obstruction. Lori will soon undergo radiation therapy to the head and spinal cord, as well as chemotherapy.

Questions 12 to 15 refer to this situation.

12 Before radiation therapy begins, the nurse should inform Lori and her parents that:

A. Her head will be marked by the radiotherapist, but these markings can be washed off after each treatment
B. She may become very drowsy during the course of treatment
C. Her blood counts will remain stable during the radiation therapy
D. Lori's parents can stay with her in the radiation treatment room

13 While receiving radiation therapy, Lori must take dexamethasone (Decadron) to prevent cerebral edema. Which side effects of this steroid medication are most common?

A. Mood changes, sodium retention, and hypertension
B. Anemia, hypotension, and decreased appetite
C. Bone marrow suppression and weight loss
D. Petechiae and immunosuppression

14 Lori develops a red, peeling area on her scalp while undergoing radiation therapy. The nurse should advise her to:

A. Wash the affected area with soap and water
B. Cover the affected area with a moist compress three times a day
C. Gently debride the area with a soft cloth soaked in a sterile saline solution
D. Apply vitamin A & D ointment immediately after radiation treatments

15 Lori asks why complete blood counts are needed once or twice a week while she receives radiation therapy. The nurse correctly explains that:

A. Radiation therapy to a large area destroys circulating red blood cells
B. Radiation therapy to a large area destroys developing bone-marrow cells
C. Radiation therapy affects platelets more than any other type of cell
D. Radiation therapy can cause a second tumor to develop

SITUATION

Tom Millhouse, age 3, is undergoing treatment for neuroblastoma. He has a central venous (Broviac) catheter in place and receives total parenteral nutrition at home for 12 hours each night.

Questions 16 to 19 refer to this situation.

16 Which complication poses the greatest threat to a patient with a central venous line, such as a Broviac or Hickman catheter?

A. Uncontrolled bleeding
B. Infection
C. Blood clot formation at the catheter tip
D. Allergic reaction

17 After discharge, Tom's dressings over the central line exit site should be changed:

A. At least twice weekly
B. Only when soiled
C. Only by the home health nurse
D. Only at clinic visits

18 Which values should the nurse monitor while Tom is undergoing treatment?

A. Serum glucose levels
B. Serum protein levels
C. Serum electrolyte levels and chemistry studies
D. All of the above

19 The nurse should advise Tom's parents to call the physician if Tom has:

A. An increased temperature that lasts longer than 24 hours
B. An increased temperature
C. An increased temperature that does not respond to acetaminophen
D. An increased temperature that is not accompanied by a cold or flu symptoms

SITUATION

David Warner, age 7, arrives at the pediatric clinic with his parents, who report a 1-week history of diplopia, facial weakness, and difficulty walking. David is admitted to the hospital for testing.

Questions 20 to 22 refer to this situation.

20 The physician orders several tests, including magnetic resonance imaging (MRI). The nurse should explain to David's parents that MRI:

A. Requires injection of radioactive material
B. Uses only a small amount of radiation, less than that of a chest X-ray
C. Visualizes bony details and calcifications
D. Uses radiofrequencies to produce computer images of internal tissues

21 David is diagnosed as having a brain stem glioma, a malignant tumor infiltrating the pons. All of the following statements about pediatric brain tumors are true *except:*

A. Brain tumors are the second leading cause of pediatric cancers and the most common type of solid tumor in children
B. Approximately 60% of childhood brain tumors arise in the posterior fossa
C. Central nervous system (CNS) tumors are most common in children ages 5 to 10
D. No contributing factors have been identified for CNS tumors

22 After several months, David's condition deteriorates despite radiation therapy. The physician and the outpatient nurse discuss terminal care with David's parents, who express a desire to have David remain at home to die. The nurse is aware that hospice care is available in the community. Hospice care is based on all of the following concepts *except:*

A. Family members are the primary caregivers, supported by a team of professionals and a volunteer staff
B. The child's physical, psychological, social, and spiritual needs are considered
C. The needs of the family are as important as those of the patient
D. The grieving process can continue for a long time, so the family's care typically continues for 1 month after the child's death

---

SITUATION

Eileen Griss, age 2, was brought to the pediatrician's office by her mother, who noticed marked swelling in her daughter's abdominal area while bathing her. The pediatrician palpated the area and detected an abdominal mass. Eileen was admitted to the hospital for a radiographic workup. Ultrasound examination revealed a right renal mass, which was confirmed by computed tomography (CT) scan. The physician performed a right nephrectomy with lymph node sampling. Pathological findings indicate that Eileen has Wilms' tumor.

Questions 23 and 24 refer to this situation.

---

23 What is the primary nursing goal following a transabdominal nephrectomy?

A. To provide comfort
B. To support and reassure the parents and child
C. To provide nourishment
D. To promote adequate hydration

24 Eileen recovers quickly and will be discharged after her first course of chemotherapy. The nurse explains to Mr. and Mrs. Griss that Eileen will receive vincristine and actinomycin D in the outpatient clinic. The nurse describes the side effects of these drugs and notes that vincristine can cause constipation. Which action should Eileen's parents take if she becomes constipated?

A. Administer a pediatric enema
B. Call the physician only if constipation persists for more than 3 days
C. Encourage Eileen to drink 18 to 24 oz of prune juice each day
D. Call the physician if Eileen does not have a bowel movement according to her usual schedule

---

SITUATION

Ron, age 14, is brought to the emergency department after sustaining an injury during a football game. He complains of pain, warmth, and swelling of the left distal femur. Radiographic studies suggest a possibile malignant bone tumor. Ron is admitted to the hospital for further evaluation and pain control. After performing extensive studies, the physician tentatively diagnoses osteosarcoma.

Questions 25 to 28 refer to this situation.

25 The physician orders a chest X-ray for Ron to:

A. Rule out the possibility of chest injury
B. Rule out metastasis to the lungs
C. Rule out metastasis to the ribs
D. Provide a baseline for anesthesia

26 The physician orders a serum alkaline phosphatase evaluation for Ron. Elevation in this value may indicate:

A. Osteoblastic activity within the tumor
B. Increased activity in the mitochondria
C. Isoenzyme activity within the bone
D. All of the above

27 Further testing confirms the tentative diagnosis of osteosarcoma. Ron's treatment plan includes preoperative chemotherapy consisting of high-dose methotrexate (HDMTX) and citrovorum factor (leucovorin). Leucovorin is used to:

A. Prevent peripheral neuropathies
B. Supplement the vitamin B_6 depleted by HDMTX
C. Rescue healthy cells from the lethal effects of HDMTX
D. Prevent HDMTX from causing sterility

28 Nursing management of a patient receiving HDMTX is directed toward all of the following *except:*

A. Maintaining strict intake and output measurements
B. Administering leucovorin simultaneously with HDMTX, as prescribed
C. Inspecting the mouth daily for signs of ulceration
D. Administering antiemetics on a regular schedule

SITUATION

Jeanne Egland, age 3, is admitted to the hospital with weakness, pallor, irritability, and weight loss. The nurse notes exophthalmos and periorbital edema. After extensive testing, the physician diag-

noses neuroblastoma stage III. Jeanne is scheduled for a cranio-tomy.

Questions 29 and 30 refer to this situation.

29 The nurse should consider which strategy when preparing Jeanne for surgery?

A. Communicating directly with Mr. and Mrs. Egland because they will be concerned about Jeanne's long-term prognosis and Jeanne is too young to understand
B. Talking with Jeanne and showing her pictures of the brain and the tumor at various stages
C. Asking Jeanne to draw the brain, then clarifying any misconceptions
D. Explaining the procedure to Jeanne at least 2 days before surgery, so she has time to understand the information

30 The nurse prepares for Jeanne's return from surgery. Which nursing intervention indicates a thorough understanding of potential postoperative problems?

A. Placing a cooling blanket on the bed
B. Placing the bed in the Trendelenburg position
C. Placing an emergency tracheostomy set at the bedside
D. Placing a commode near the bed

SITUATION

Sam Williams, age 6, was diagnosed with acute myeloblastic leukemia (AML) at age 2. Throughout the course of the illness, the nursing staff has established a therapeutic relationship with the entire family.

Several months ago, Sam was readmitted to the hospital because of a relapse. Attempts to achieve remission failed, and Mr. and Mrs. Williams have been told that he will die soon.

Questions 31 to 37 refer to this situation.

31 Mrs. Williams's conversations with the nurse focus on her memories of happier times. She frequently cries and asks, "Why did this have to happen?" This behavior can best be described as:

A. Despair
B. Anticipatory grief
C. Bargaining
D. Grief resolution

32 Mr. and Mrs. Williams ask the nurse if they should tell Sam that he is dying. In helping the parents reach a decision, the nurse replies:

A. "In my experience, telling a child that he is dying causes too much anxiety"
B. "Only a child over age 10 can understand that he is dying, so Sam will not benefit from being told"
C. "Most studies show that children should be protected from the knowledge that they are dying"
D. "Being honest with Sam promotes an atmosphere in which thoughts and feelings can be shared"

33 In preparing a nursing care plan, the most important factor to understand is Sam's:

A. Past experiences with death and dying
B. Religious beliefs
C. Understanding of death in relation to his growth and development
D. Feelings toward his parents

34 Which is the most effective way to assess Sam's level of understanding about death and dying?

A. Directly questioning him about his thoughts on death
B. Providing opportunities for nonverbal communication, such as through puppetry and drawing
C. Role playing with Sam and his parents
D. All of the above

35 Lauren, Sam's 3-year-old sister, is playing with her dolls. The nurse overhears her say, "Molly, you're dead, but remember to be home at 5 o'clock for dinner." This conversation is:

A. Unnatural and morbid
B. Indicative of the child's sense of humor
C. Bordering on a psychotic response to her brother's illness
D. Within normal limits of behavior for a 3-year-old child

36 Mr. and Mrs. Williams ask for advice about joining a self-help support group for the bereaved, such as Compassionate Friends. Based on her knowledge, the nurse should reply:

A. "Professional therapy is more beneficial than a self-help group"
B. "Support groups fill a need for those who want to share their feelings with others"
C. "Support groups encourage persons to grieve for a prolonged period of time"
D. "Attending a support group meeting would not be helpful"

37 Ten months after Sam's death, Mrs. Williams reports to a visiting nurse that Claude, Sam's 11-year-old brother, has become aggressive and is having trouble sleeping. The nurse should:

A. Gather more information about the child's behavior
B. Refer the child to a psychologist specializing in grief and loss
C. Reassure Mrs. Williams that her child is just going through a preadolescent stage
D. Tell Mrs. Williams that these behaviors probably are symptoms of school problems

Answer sheet

	A B C D		A B C D
1	○ ○ ○ ○	31	○ ○ ○ ○
2	○ ○ ○ ○	32	○ ○ ○ ○
3	○ ○ ○ ○	33	○ ○ ○ ○
4	○ ○ ○ ○	34	○ ○ ○ ○
5	○ ○ ○ ○	35	○ ○ ○ ○
6	○ ○ ○ ○	36	○ ○ ○ ○
7	○ ○ ○ ○	37	○ ○ ○ ○
8	○ ○ ○ ○		
9	○ ○ ○ ○		
10	○ ○ ○ ○		
11	○ ○ ○ ○		
12	○ ○ ○ ○		
13	○ ○ ○ ○		
14	○ ○ ○ ○		
15	○ ○ ○ ○		
16	○ ○ ○ ○		
17	○ ○ ○ ○		
18	○ ○ ○ ○		
19	○ ○ ○ ○		
20	○ ○ ○ ○		
21	○ ○ ○ ○		
22	○ ○ ○ ○		
23	○ ○ ○ ○		
24	○ ○ ○ ○		
25	○ ○ ○ ○		
26	○ ○ ○ ○		
27	○ ○ ○ ○		
28	○ ○ ○ ○		
29	○ ○ ○ ○		
30	○ ○ ○ ○		

Answers and rationales

1 Correct answer—**A**

In leukemia, leukemic blast cells proliferate in the bone marrow and replace functioning white blood cells. Because they are immature, these cells are incapable of fighting infection. Consequently, Jerome is at increased risk for infection because of his decreased number of functioning white blood cells. Limiting environmental stimulation is not necessary from a medical standpoint, although it may minimize overall stress. Proper nutrition is important, but it is not critical at this time. Death is not imminent in this situation; therefore, determining the child's concept of death is not a priority.

2 Correct answer—**D**

Although straining at defecation is contraindicated in a thrombocytopenic patient because of the risk of intracranial and rectal bleeding, introducing a suppository into the delicate rectal mucosa can cause small tears. This would place a neutropenic patient at increased risk for infection. Limiting the number of venipunctures is appropriate because they are potential sites of infection. Taking rectal temperatures should be avoided because the thermometer can traumatize the rectal mucosa and cause bleeding or infection. A child whose platelet count is low should limit his activities to prevent injury and subsequent hemorrhage.

3 Correct answer—**B**

Initial treatment for a child with leukemia begins with administration of steroids, usually prednisone. Because prednisone therapy tends to increase a patient's appetite, encouraging Jerome's food intake is unnecessary. Prednisone may cause fluid retention; therefore, the nurse should monitor Jerome's sodium intake and weigh him daily to determine whether fluids are being retained. Frequent blood pressure checks also are necessary because fluid retention may cause hypertension.

4 Correct answer—**B**

Lymphoblasts usually respond well to chemotherapy, and tumor cell lysis can be expected soon after chemotherapy is initiated. The lysis of a large number of cells releases substantial amounts of uric acid, which can accumulate and precipitate in the kidney, causing tubular obstruction. Allopurinol prevents hyperuricemic nephropathy by inhibiting the enzyme necessary for uric acid production. Alkalinization of the urine helps to prevent uric acid formation. Allupurinol has no cytotoxic properties and therefore does not contribute to tumor lysis. Doxorubicin damages cardiac tissue, not the kidney.

5 Correct answer—C

The family of a child who is newly diagnosed with cancer may have altered perceptions and a decreased ability to learn. Therefore, the nurse should keep explanations on a basic level and begin teaching before the child is discharged. Parents should be able to recognize the side effects of treatment and know how to manage them. They also must be able to recognize the signs and symptoms of infection and bleeding and know how to respond when these problems occur. Withholding information from the parents is inadvisable. The nurse should disclose any information she can to establish a trusting relationship with the family. She should limit the teaching to short sessions and keep in mind that she may need to repeat this information many times throughout the child's treatment. She should encourage family members to write down their questions so that they will not forget them. Pamphlets and booklets may overwhelm the family at first; the nurse can supplement her teaching with them later.

6 Correct answer—D

Although a child may experience growth problems related to childhood cancer, he typically catches up when treatment is discontinued. Growth-limiting effects of radiation depend on the child's age and the radiation dosage. Administering radiation during rapid growth periods, such as early childhood and puberty, significantly affects growth. Regardless of age, radiation doses greater than 2,000 rads adversely affect growth. An endocrinologic consultation is indicated for any child who does not grow normally after radiation is discontinued. A child's growth disturbances may be related to growth hormone deficiency or thyroid dysfunction, which warrants assessment of these hormones. Wrist X-rays are commonly obtained to evaluate the child's skeletal maturity, which may or may not coincide with his chronological age. Growth-hormone injections are given only after the workup is completed and a growth-hormone deficiency is diagnosed.

7 Correct answer—**D**

Approximately 60% of children who are currently diagnosed with cancer will be long-term survivors. By the year 2000, one of every 900 adults between ages 20 and 29 will be a survivor of childhood cancer. Use of the three modalities of treatment (surgery, chemotherapy, and radiation) has improved the survival rate of children with cancer. Combination chemotherapy (such as those agents used to treat leukemia) also has had a positive effect. Patients with osteosarcoma have reaped enormous benefits from adjuvant chemotherapy. Previously, amputation was the primary method of treatment for this type of cancer, and the survival rate was about 25% in 1970. The use of adjuvant chemotherapy has increased the survival rate in these patients to about 70%. Clinical trials provide valuable information about the treatment of childhood cancers; this knowledge has helped improve survival rates for pediatric oncology patients.

8 Correct answer—**D**

Childhood cancer and its treatment can generate many potential delayed effects. The type and degree of these effects depend on the amount and type of therapy, as well as the child's age at the time of treatment. Survivors of childhood cancer are at increased risk for secondary cancers, with a peak occurrence 3 to 6 years after therapy is discontinued. In addition to the central nervous system and endocrine effects that may be observed in survivors of leukemia, other long-term effects may include cardiac toxicity in response to anthracycline administration and liver damage associated with methotrexate and 6-mercaptopurine therapy. Continued immunosuppression is not a concern for patients after therapy is stopped. Although keeping records up to date is essential during the acute stage of illness, it is not as important during follow-up treatment, especially since Bill has been in remission for several years. Any side effects of treatment would have dissipated by now; the nurse should be monitoring for latent effects, not side effects, of Bill's treatment.

9 Correct answer—**B**

Hodgkin's disease is a cancer of the lymphoid system that primarily affects the lymph nodes but can metastasize to the spleen, liver, bone marrow, and lungs. At diagnosis, the disease is staged from I to IV, with stage I being the most limited and stage IV the most extensive. The stages are further subdivided into A and B, with A being the absence of generalized symptoms and B being the presence of generalized symptoms. Fever, weight loss, and night sweats are three signs of Hodgkin's disease stage B. Additional general symptoms include anorexia, nausea, and pruritis. Hepatomegaly, splenomegaly, and lymph node size influence the determination of stages I through IV. Malaise is a common side effect of radiation treatment.

10 Correct answer—C

The nurse should consider the treatment plan when selecting the appropriate venous access device. For example, indwelling ports are designed for intermittent use. An external device, such as a Broviac or Hickman catheter, may be more appropriate than a subcutaneous device, such as a Port-a-Cath, for frequent access. However, even though the skin must be punctured each time a subcutaneous device is accessed, this type of device does not require dressings and allows for swimming and bathing. It is also inconspicuous and has less of an impact on the child's body image. Neither the size of the child nor the size of the veins influences the type of device. The surgeon's preference also is not a factor.

11 Correct answer—B

To ensure compliance, the nurse should try to conform Danielle's medication schedule to an adolescent's life-style. Danielle will not want to take medication during after-school activities when she is with her friends. Recommending that she take her medication with meals or during routine hygiene regimens minimizes life-style disruptions. Also, pairing administration with particular activities serves as a reminder to take the medications. Danielle should be aware of the potential side effects of her medication and know which effects to report to her physician.

12 Correct answer—B

Patients commonly complain of drowsiness (somnolence syndrome) during or within a few weeks after receiving radiation therapy. The cause of this drowsiness is unknown. The radiotherapist's markings are used as guidelines for the radiation treatment and should not be washed off. Because bone marrow suppression is a side effect of radiation therapy, the parent's should be told that Lori's blood counts will decrease. Parents are not permitted in the radiation room while treatment is administered.

13 Correct answer—A

Dexamethasone's side effects include mood changes, sodium retention, hypertension, increased appetite, and weight gain; these effects are dose-dependent. Although immunosuppression is a side effect of this drug, petechiae are not.

14 Correct answer—D

A patient who develops cutaneous reactions to radiation therapy should not use soap or lotions containing alcohol or perfumes because these agents can dry the affected area and lead to further excoriation, skin breakdown, and infection. A bland, hydrophilic lotion, such as vitamin A & D ointment, may be ordered.

15 Correct answer—B

Although most white cells, red cells, and platelets are not adversely affected by radiation therapy, the precursors of these cells, located in the bone marrow, are extremely sensitive to radiation treatment. A patient's peripheral blood count drops as the number of bone marrow cells decreases; this effect is especially noticeable if the radiation field encompasses a large area of bone marrow. Thus, complete blood counts are needed once or twice a week during radiation therapy to monitor for low levels of white cells, red cells, and platelets. Patients with low red blood cell counts commonly receive transfusions of packed red cells. Radiation therapy is sometimes responsible for second tumors; however, this response is delayed and would not be detected by a complete blood count.

16 Correct answer—B

The tip of a central venous line rests in the right atrium of the heart. The other end of the catheter is tunneled under the skin to an exit site on the chest. The placement of the catheter, the care that is required, and the immunosuppressive effects of chemotherapy all contribute to an increased risk of infection. Thus, systemic infection is the greatest threat to a cancer patient with a central venous line in place. Although uncontrolled bleeding is not a common problem, blood that leaks from the catheter can be managed by clamping the area between the leak and the catheter exit site. Regular flushing of the catheter line prevents blood clot formation. Allergic reactions usually are not associated with use of a central venous line catheter.

17 Correct answer—A

Although they may be initially reluctant, parents and children quickly learn how to care for central lines. If not cleaned regularly, the exit site of the catheter can become infected. Once the infection spreads to the subcutaneous tissue, it is difficult to treat. Therefore, the exit site should be cleaned at least twice weekly with alcohol, followed by application of an appropriate solution (most institutions use povidone-iodine) and ointment. The area should then be covered with a sterile dressing or bandage; if the dressing becomes wet or soiled, it should be changed immediately.

18 Correct answer—D

The nurse must monitor the patient's serum glucose, protein, and electrolyte levels and chemistry studies because of the side effects of total parenteral nutrition (TPN). The high-dextrose solution used for TPN necessitates monitoring of serum glucose levels. Protein levels are monitored to assess the effects of TPN on the patient's nutritional status. Serum electrolytes and chemistry studies are checked because TPN can damage a patient's liver and pancreas.

19 Correct answer—B

Sepsis can develop rapidly in an immunocompromised child. Therefore, the nurse should advise the parents to call the physician immediately if Tom experiences any increase in temperature—this may be the first, or only, sign of sepsis.

20 Correct answer—D

Magnetic resonance imaging (MRI) uses radiofrequency emissions from elements, particularly hydrogen, to produce computer images of internal tissues. A strong magnetic field changes the orientation of these elements within the body; the image then is recorded and converted to a computerized picture. MRI is a noninvasive procedure that does not involve injection of radioactive material or the use of radiation. It permits visualization of morphologic features and tissue discrimination but does not show bony details or calcifications.

21 Correct answer—D

Although the etiology of brain tumors is unknown, some contributing factors have been identified, including exposure to radiation and the presence of immunologic disorders, such as neurofibromatosis and tuberous sclerosis. Brain tumors are the second most common form of cancer in children (leukemia is the most common). Most brain tumors in children arise in the posterior fossa; in adults, brain tumors are more likely to appear in the anterior portion of the brain. Central nervous system tumors are most common in children between ages 5 and 10.

22 Correct answer—D

Many hospice programs contact families for several years, not just for 1 month, after the death of a loved one. The patient's comfort is the principal consideration in hospice care. Family members are the primary caregivers, but they are supported by professionals and volunteers. Hospice care addresses the physical, psychological, social, and spiritual needs of the patient and his family. The needs of the family members and of the patient are of equal importance. The concepts of hospice care can be employed in a home setting or a hospice care facility.

23 Correct answer—D

Although providing comfort, reassurance, and nourishment are important, promoting adequate hydration is the primary nursing goal for a patient who has undergone a transabdominal nephrectomy; adequate hydration helps maintain fluid balance and proper kidney function.

24 Correct answer—D

Vincristine (Oncovin) is a plant alkaloid that arrests mitosis at metaphase and inhibits cell division. The drug's chief adverse effect is neurotoxicity. Paralytic ileus, beginning as constipation, also may occur. Therefore, the parents should notify the physician if the child does not have bowel movements according to her usual schedule. Home remedies, such as administering enemas or ingesting prune juice, would be ineffective in this case; the constipation is caused by lack of peristalsis, not obstruction.

25 Correct answer—B

Osteosarcoma generally metastasizes to the lungs before moving to other sites. Therefore, the physician orders chest X-rays at the time of diagnosis to determine whether pulmonary metastasis has occurred. Chest injury is not a factor in osteosarcoma. This type of cancer metastasizes to the lungs, not the ribs. A chest X-ray is performed for diagnostic purposes, not as a baseline for anesthesia.

26 Correct answer—A

Osteosarcoma arises from bone-forming cells. An increased level of alkaline phosphatase, a substance normally found in developing bone, may indicate osteoblastic (bone-forming) activity within the tumor. This simple test also may be used to measure a patient's response to treatment. Mitochondria are involved in protein synthesis and lipid metabolism. Isoenzyme studies help to determine cardiac muscle, not osteoblastic, activity.

27 Correct answer—C

Leucovorin calcium is administered as an antidote to high-dose methotrexate therapy (HDMTX). Leucovorin competes with the methotrexate for entrance into healthy cells and "rescues" them from the potentially lethal effects of the drug. Methotrexate cannot penetrate a cell that has already been entered by leucovorin. HDMTX does not cause peripheral neuropathies or sterility nor does it deplete vitamin B_6 stores.

28 Correct answer—B

Leucovorin is administered after HDMTX therapy has been completed. If the drugs are given simultaneously, leucovorin interferes with the cytotoxic effects of HDMTX. A patient receiving HDMTX is given large amounts of I.V. fluids to prevent nephrotoxicity. Strict intake and output measurements are essential because decreased urine output may indicate nephrotoxicity. Mouth ulcers are a sign of HDMTX toxicity, meaning that the drug has affected normal cells in addition to malignant ones. Premedication and administration of antiemetics on a regular schedule help to prevent nausea and vomiting.

29 Correct answer—C

The first step in preparing Jeanne for surgery is to assess her knowledge level. By asking Jeanne to draw the brain, the nurse can base her teaching on the child's level of understanding. A 3-year-old child should be involved in preoperative preparation. However, explaining the staging of the tumor and actual brain anatomy to the child is too sophisticated. Preschoolers have a limited concept of time, so the nurse should explain the procedure shortly or immediately before the surgery.

30 Correct answer—A

Temperature swings are common postoperatively. Placing a cooling blanket on the bed before the child returns is an excellent way to prepare for the possibility of fever. Patient positioning after a craniotomy is critical but usually is determined by the surgeon. The Trendelenburg position, however, is contraindicated in all types of cranial surgery because it increases intracranial pressure and the risk of hemorrhage. Respiratory infections commonly develop in patients undergoing craniotomy as a result of atelectasis or aspiration, but not obstruction. Therefore, the appropriate treatment involves administration of antibiotics, not an emergency tracheostomy. Fluids are closely monitored postoperatively because of the increased risk of fluid retention. Diuretics, such as mannitol or dextrose, may be administered to produce rapid diuresis. Urine output is monitored by catheterization to assess the effectiveness of the diuretics. A commode is unnecessary because the patient has a catheter in place.

31 Correct answer—B

The grief process usually begins during the terminal phase of an illness, before a child actually dies. Anticipatory grief is described as an inner process of acknowledging, managing, and coming to terms with the loss of a relationship. Parents may have a strong need to talk about their child, review his life, and imagine what it will be like without him. Despair typically occurs after the death of a loved one, when the individual experiences emptiness and feels that life has no meaning. Bargaining is characterized as an attempt to postpone the inevitable. Grief resolution is the final outcome of the grieving process.

32 Correct answer—D

Based on her extensive research on death and dying, Elisabeth Kübler-Ross determined that the question is not whether to tell a person that he is dying but rather how to tell him. Studies by Spinetta and Maloney, as well as by Waechter, conclude that developing a trusting atmosphere is important. If the parents are honest with the child about his condition, the child and his significant others can express their positive and negative feelings and offset their feelings of denial. The child's remaining time should be spent effectively, and emotional energy should not be wasted by pretending that everything is fine.

33 Correct answer—C

To plan appropriate care, the nurse must understand the patient's developmental level and his perspective on death. Although Sam's experiences and religious beliefs are significant, the most important factor is his level of understanding and concept of death. Children typically are fearful about the impact that their death will have on others. The nurse can begin discussions about his feelings toward his parents after assessing his perspective and level of understanding.

34 Correct answer—B

Even in an atmosphere in which communication is encouraged, many children have difficulty expressing their feelings, especially negative ones of fear, separation, and punishment. Examining nonverbal cues during play provides a valuable source of information for the nurse. More direct methods of eliciting information may be too threatening to a young child.

35 Correct answer—D

Preschoolers are generally more comfortable expressing their feelings during play. Although children age 3 recognize that things end, they do not understand the finality of death. They commonly believe that dead persons continue to eat, walk, and play.

36 Correct answer—B

Self-help support groups provide grieving parents with a safe, comforting atmosphere in which to share their thoughts, feelings, anger, and pain. Exchanging information, affirming that their reactions are appropriate, and sharing memories of the lost child help in the healing process. Meeting with parents who have coped with their child's death and gone on with their lives can help Mr. and Mrs. Williams look forward to the future. No evidence indicates that professional therapy is more beneficial than self-help support groups. Self-help support groups do not promote prolonged grieving.

37 Correct answer—A

Children grieve in various ways. Their expressions of grief are commonly different from those of an adult; somatic complaints, sleep anxieties, aggression, and misbehavior are common grieving reactions in children. The nurse needs more information about the child's behavior before making an appropriate recommendation.

CHAPTER 10

Emotional and
Psychological
Problems

Questions

1 Anxiety in a school-age child usually is related to:

   A. Bodily injury and mutilation
   B. Social relationships
   C. Death and dying
   D. Family relationships

2 What is the best way to manage school phobia?

   A. Return the child to school
   B. Allow the child to avoid school temporarily
   C. Allow the child a prolonged absence from school
   D. Seek a home tutor for the child

3 Enuresis commonly results from:

   A. Severe emotional disturbances
   B. Parental problems in child rearing
   C. Familial tendencies
   D. Nightmares

4 Which symptom is characteristic of childhood depression?

   A. Bulimia
   B. Inability to concentrate
   C. Anxiety
   D. Irritability

5 Schizophrenia in a child differs from that in an adult with respect to:

   A. Onset
   B. Defense mechanisms
   C. Reality orientation
   D. Symptoms

6 Autism is a condition usually associated with:

   A. Boys
   B. Girls
   C. Hearing deficits
   D. A high IQ

SITUATION

Dolores, age 13, swallows thirty 325-mg tablets of acetaminophen after an argument with her mother. About 4 hours later, Dolores tells her mother about swallowing the tablets. At the emergency department, Dolores's acetaminophen level is 180 mcg/ml. Dolores is admitted to the pediatric unit for overdose treatment and evaluation of her suicide attempt.

Questions 7 to 12 refer to this situation.

7 Which phase of acetaminophen toxicity is deceptive because of its latent presentation?

  A. Phase I
. **B.** Phase II
  C. Phase III
  D. None of the above

8 Lethargy and coma during the first 24 hours after acetaminophen toxicity indicate:

  A. A large overdose of acetaminophen
  B. The patient is in phase 1 of toxicity
  C. Another drug has been ingested
  D. Immediate induction of emesis is necessary

9 Which is the treatment of choice for Dolores?

  A. Induced emesis or lavage and supportive fluid therapy
  B. Induced emesis or lavage and activated charcoal
  C. Induced emesis or lavage and N-acetylcysteine (NAC)
  D. Induced emesis or lavage, activated charcoal, and NAC

10 Which statement about adolescent suicide is *true?*

  A. Adolescents who discuss suicide do not follow through
  B. Many suicidal adolescents give clues to their intention
  C. Adolescent boys attempt suicide more often than adolescent girls
  D. A suicidal adolescent is suicidal for life

11 Which approach is most effective in gathering information about Dolores's suicidal intent?

A. Directly questioning Dolores
B. Indirectly questioning Dolores
C. Questioning Dolores's family
D. Observing Dolores's behavior

12 Dolores tells the nurse that she feels depressed, hopeless, and isolated. Which nursing action can help decrease Dolores's feelings of hopelessness and isolation?

A. Promoting extreme cheerfulness
B. Providing oppportunties for Dolores to express her feelings
C. Avoiding setting limits
D. None of the above

SITUATION

Brad, age 16, is brought to the emergency department by two of his friends. The nurse notes that he is agitated and pacing, and his speech is becoming increasingly incoherent. He begs the nurse to protect him because "The gang is after me and they are going to kill me." According to his friends, Brad has been snorting cocaine every 10 minutes for the past several hours.

Questions 13 to 15 refer to this situation.

13 Which vital sign readings are consistent with a repeated intake of cocaine?

A. Blood pressure, 120/80 mm Hg; pulse rate, 84 beats/minute; respirations, 12 breaths/minute
B. Blood pressure, 160/100 mm Hg; pulse rate, 116 beats/minute; respirations, 22 breaths/minute
C. Blood pressure, 140/90 mm Hg; pulse rate, 86 beats/minute; respirations, 16 breaths/minute
D. Blood pressure, 110/70 mm Hg; pulse rate, 72 beats/minute; respirations, 10 breaths/minute

14 When Brad began snorting cocaine earlier in the day, he probably exhibited:

A. Laughter, excitement, and hyperactivity
B. Drowsiness, decreased activity, and slowed speech
C. Angry outbursts, slurred speech, and unsteady gait
D. Confusion, fear of strangers, and compulsive eating

15 When the cocaine's effects wear off, Brad probably will experience:

A. Anger
B. Depression
C. Mania
D. Forgetfulness

SITUATION

Shelly Clarke, age 14, is admitted to the adolescent unit of the hospital following a car accident in which her mother was driving. Shelly suffered a concussion, a fractured femur, and serious hand lacerations. During the nursing history, the nurse asks about drug and alcohol use. Shelly does not make eye contact with the nurse and answers evasively, "I don't drink any more than some other people in my family."

Questions 16 to 19 refer to this situation.

16 What is the best way for the nurse to assess Shelly's use of alcohol?

A. Refer Shelly to her physician
B. Ask Shelly's parents if they suspect that she has been drinking
C. Ask Shelly to specify how much and how often she drinks
D. Ask Shelly if she drinks when she is alone or with other people

17 The nurse suspects that Shelly may be trying to tell her that misuse of alcohol is a problem in the Clarke family. The best way for the nurse to pursue this issue is to:

A. Confront Shelly's parents and ask if either or both of them are alcoholic
B. Inform Shelly that every family has different habits regarding alcohol use and ask her to describe her family's habits
C. Promise not to tell Shelly's parents if she describes their drinking habits
D. Inform Shelly that her parents are adults and that most adults use alcohol socially

18 Shelly tells the nurse that she does not drink every day, never drinks in the morning, and never drinks anything stronger than beer or wine. She is sure that she does not have a problem with alcohol. How should the nurse respond?

A. "Well, that's good. I guess you don't have anything to worry about then"
B. "You really shouldn't drink at all at your age"
C. "Just because you don't drink every day doesn't mean you aren't an alcoholic"
D. "The alcohol content in beer and wine is the same as that in hard liquor, and not everyone who has a problem with alcohol drinks every day or in the morning"

19 Which statement about alcohol abuse among women is *true?*

A. Women who abuse alcohol do not usually become alcoholic
B. Women who abuse alcohol are less likely to hide their drinking
C. Women with drinking problems are found in every age-group, socioeconomic class, racial or ethnic group, and employment situation
D. All of the above

SITUATION

Barbara, age 15, comes to the mental health clinic seeking help. During the nursing history, the nurse learns that Barbara has been taking over-the-counter diet pills to help her lose weight. She also has been dieting, drinking large quantities of black coffee during the day, and drinking alcohol at night to help her sleep. She recently began acquiring a supply of diazepam (Valium) from someone at school to help her calm down.

Questions 20 to 23 refer to this situation.

20 Barbara's anxiety and difficulty sleeping are probably the result of:

A. Abuse of diet pills and caffeine
B. Inappropriate use of diazepam
C. Stringent dieting and worrying about her weight
D. Alcohol use

21 Which question is most effective in eliciting information about Barbara's use of drugs and alcohol?

A. "Why are you trying to lose weight when you are already so thin?"
B. "Are you worrying about anything in particular that is causing you to use drugs and alcohol in this way?"
C. "Do your parents know that you have been taking drugs and alcohol?"
D. "Will you tell me exactly which drugs you have been taking, how much you have been drinking, and how long you have been doing this?"

22 The combined use of alcohol and diazepam is particularly dangerous because:

A. Alcohol and diazepam are antagonists
B. Alcohol and diazepam are both central nervous system depressants
C. Alcohol and diazepam are cardiac irritants when taken in combination
D. Alcohol and diazepam produce severe anxiety when taken in combination

23 In planning Barbara's care, the nurse's first consideration should be to:

A. Instruct Barbara about the effects of drugs and alcohol on her body and the dangers of multiple drug use
B. Teach Barbara relaxation techniques for more effective stress management
C. Determine Barbara's knowledge of nutrition and help her to plan an effective weight-loss program
D. Determine Barbara's level of drug and alcohol abuse and whether she requires detoxification

Answer sheet

A B C D

1 ○○○○
2 ○○○○
3 ○○○○
4 ○○○○
5 ○○○○
6 ○○○○
7 ○○○○
8 ○○○○
9 ○○○○
10 ○○○○
11 ○○○○
12 ○○○○
13 ○○○○
14 ○○○○
15 ○○○○
16 ○○○○
17 ○○○○
18 ○○○○
19 ○○○○
20 ○○○○
21 ○○○○
22 ○○○○
23 ○○○○

Answers and rationales

1 Correct answer—**B**

A school-age child typically is becoming more involved in the community and school and beginning to develop social relationships. Friends are the primary focus at this time. A school-age child tends to worry less than a preschooler about body intactness and family relationships. Such a child also does not tend to worry about death unless faced with a serious illness.

2 Correct answer—**A**

A child with school phobia may feel threatened at school (for example, because of contact with a bully, a gang, or an overly critical teacher) or have a fear of examinations. The child also may fear leaving home. The best therapy is to return the child to school immediately; this action will increase his self-worth and esteem. Permitting the child to avoid school temporarily or allowing a prolonged absence from school significantly increases the difficulty of initiating regular school attendance. Using a home tutor allows the child to avoid the problem and reaffirms his perceived inability to cope with the situation. If the phobia results from a real threat from a bully or teacher, the matter should be handled accordingly; however, the child should attend school while a solution to the problem is sought.

3 Correct answer—**C**

Enuresis—repeated involuntary urination in a child who is beyond the age when bladder control should have been established—is associated with a familial tendency toward bed wetting. It is more common in boys than girls. Enuresis is not caused by emotional disorders, problems with child-rearing practices, or nightmares.

4 Correct answer—**B**

Childhood depression is manifested by sleep disturbances, poor appetite, inability to concentrate, decreased ability to think, low energy, and apathy. If symptoms persist for more than 2 weeks, psychotherapy may be necessary.

5 Correct answer—**A**

Schizophrenia is a group of mental disorders characterized by disturbances in thinking, mood, and behavior. A schizophrenic person has an altered concept of reality that may include hallucinations and delusions. Mood changes, inappropriate affect, and withdrawn, aggressive, or bizarre behavior are additional signs of this disorder. The symptoms of childhood schizophrenia occur gradually, while those of adult schizophrenia have an abrupt onset. Both children and adults with schizophrenia use defense mechanisms and display disturbed reality orientation. Symptoms of schizophrenia do not differ according to the age of the patient.

6 Correct answer—**A**

Autism is a complex developmental disorder marked by severe intellectual and behavioral deficits. Autistic children display unusual, often repetitive, behaviors; they are unresponsive to social relationships, speak in peculiar language, and have altered sensory-perceptual processing. The prognosis usually is poor; most autistic children require life-long supervision and assistance. Autism is four times more common in boys than girls. Although autistic children may act as if they have a hearing deficit, their hearing usually is intact. Most of these children are retarded and have IQs of less than 52.

7 Correct answer—**B**

Phase II of acetaminophen toxicity (latent period) occurs 24 to 36 hours postingestion and is characterized by a disappearance of the patient's symptoms. The patient and her family should be prepared for this event, so they do not assume that the patient has recovered. During phase I (the first 24 hours after ingestion), the patient may experience malaise, pallor, diaphoresis, anorexia, nausea, and vomiting. In phase III (3 to 5 days after ingestion), the earlier symptoms may recur, mild jaundice may develop, and the liver may enlarge.

8 Correct answer—**C**

The symptoms of phase I acetaminophen toxicity (malaise, pallor, diaphoresis, anorexia, nausea, and vomiting) occur regardless of the amount of drug ingested. If lethargy and coma occur, ingestion of another drug should be suspected. Induction of emesis is contraindicated in a lethargic or comatose patient because of the possibility of aspiration.

9 Correct answer—C

The treatment of choice in this situation is induced emesis or lavage, followed by 20% N-acetylcysteine (NAC). Ideally, this treatment should take place within the first 10 hours after ingestion. NAC is given if treatment is delayed for more than 2 hours after the overdose; it protects the liver by binding with the acetaminophen metabolite. Activated charcoal is used if treatment is administered within the first 2 hours or if other toxins are ingested. Either NAC or activated charcoal may used, but not together. Supportive fluid therapy is insufficient to prevent toxicity.

10 Correct answer—B

Many suicidal persons, including adolescents, give clues to their impending suicide attempt. They may make such statements as "You'll never see me again" or "It will all be over tomorrow." Other clues include a sudden interest in music and art with heavy death themes, giving away possessions, or asking to leave their body to science. Adolescents who state intent should always be taken seriously because they may follow through. Adolescent girls attempt suicide more often than boys, but adolescent boys are more successful in their attempts. A suicidal adolescent is not necessarily suicidal for life.

11 Correct answer—A

Direct questioning is necessary to elicit information about a patient's intent and the severity of the problem. Asking Dolores if she is suicidal will not create suicidal ideation; most patients are relieved when someone confronts them on this issue with empathy and understanding. Indirect questioning can create a feeling of mistrust. Questioning the family or relying on observations may not yield accurate information.

12 Correct answer—B

To decrease the child's feelings of hopelessness and isolation, the nurse should provide opportunities for Dolores to express her feelings. Her suicide attempt was a faulty method of conveying how she feels. Approaches that might work successfully include verbalizing and play, art, and bibliotherapy. Promoting extreme cheerfulness would be of little value because it does not encourage Dolores to discuss her feelings. Setting limits, in terms of appropriate behavior and means of expression, probably is necessary in this situation because many adolescents have not developed internal controls.

13 Correct answer—B

Cocaine is a potent vasoconstrictor. Increasing dosages of cocaine stimulate the lower centers of the brain (thalamus, hypothalamus, and reticular formation), resulting in markedly elevated blood pressure (greater than 150/90 mm Hg), pulse rate (greater than 100 beats/minute), and respirations (greater than 20 breaths/minute). Readings of 140/90 mm Hg, 86 beats/minute, and 16 breaths/minute are not high enough to be consistent with the patient's history; the blood pressure is borderline hypertensive and the pulse and respiratory rates are within normal limits. The readings in option A are normal; those in option D, depressed.

14 Correct answer—A

Because the initial stimulating effects of cocaine on the cerebral cortex result in transient euphoria, Brad probably exhibited laughter, excitement, and hyperactivity. Duration of this initial phase depends on the dose and route of administration. Peak effects occur within 3 to 5 minutes after smoking or I.V. use, 20 to 60 minutes after intranasal use, and 60 to 90 minutes after oral ingestion.

15 Correct answer—B

Cocaine dysphoria commonly follows the transient euphoria of cocaine use. The symptoms of cocaine dysphoria are similar to those of major depression, including anxiety, sadness, apathy, anorexia, and insomnia. In chronic heavy users of cocaine, the depression and dysphoria may be severe and accompanied by suicidal ideation.

16 Correct answer—C

A nursing history should always begin with a general screening question. If the patient responds affirmatively about alcohol or drug use, or responds in a cryptic manner, the nurse should ask a more specific question, such as "How many times a week do you drink alcohol?" The nurse needs to obtain more information before referring Shelly to her physician. Questioning Shelly's parents is inappropriate because they may provide incorrect information, and this approach can alienate the adolescent. Whether the patient drinks alone or with others is less important than how much and how often she drinks.

17 Correct answer—B

The nurse's objective is to obtain more information and to encourage the patient to talk. Using a nonjudgmental approach increases trust and facilitates sharing of information. Informing Shelly that families have different habits regarding alcohol use demonstrates that the nurse is willing to hear about her family and will not judge them negatively. Because most alcoholic persons deny their drinking problem when confronted, questioning Shelly's parents would be unproductive. Making a promise that the nurse may be unable to keep could destroy the adolescent's trust in the nurse. Informing Shelly that most adults drink socially may give the impression that the nurse does not believe that her parents have a drinking problem.

18 Correct answer—D

Shelly's statements indicate that she believes popular myths about alcohol use and alcoholism. Describing the alcohol content in beer and wine and discussing the characteristics of an alcoholic person relays correct information in a nonthreatening manner. Telling Shelly that she has nothing to worry about reinforces her misperceptions. Admonishing Shelly about her drinking is judgmental and should be avoided. Although the statement "Just because you don't drink every day doesn't mean you aren't an alcoholic" conveys correct information, the use of the term *alcoholic* may frighten Shelly and put her on the defensive.

19 Correct answer—C

Like men, women with alcohol problems are found in every age-group, socioeconomic class, racial and ethnic group, and employment situation. Women who abuse alcohol become alcoholic as often as men who abuse alcohol. Female alcoholics are more likely than male alcoholics to hide their drinking.

20 Correct answer—A

Many over-the-counter preparations, such as diet pills, contain central nervous system (CNS) stimulants that can contribute to anxiety and insomnia. Coffee contains caffeine, another CNS stimulant. Diazepam is a mild tranquilizer that decreases anxiety and tension. Alcohol is a CNS depressant used by some individuals to reduce anxiety and promote sleep. Although dieting and worrying can contribute to Barbara's problem, pharmacologic causes are most likely.

21 Correct answer—D

The most important information for the nurse to obtain is the type, amount, frequency, and duration of Barbara's drug and alcohol use. "Why are you trying to lose weight when you are already so thin?" is a judgmental question. Asking whether Barbara is worrying about anything in particular assumes that she is using medication to cope with psychological problems, which may not be the case. Determining whether Barbara's parents know about her drug and alcohol use does not elicit relevant information.

22 Correct answer—B

Alcohol and diazepam are both CNS depressants. When taken in combination, they can cause severe respiratory depression, coma, and death.

23 Correct answer—D

Determining the extent of Barbara's drug and alcohol abuse is the nurse's first consideration when planning further treatment. Detoxification, if necessary, depends on the type and amount of substance ingested; it involves removing the substance from the patient's system and providing supportive management of symptoms. The nurse may instruct the patient about the effects of drugs and alcohol, teach her relaxation techniques, and plan an effective weight-loss program after establishing the need for detoxification.

CHAPTER 11

Endocrine Disorders

Questions

SITUATION

Robin Quill, age 14, has been diabetic since age 10 months. Until this past year, his condition was well-controlled by his parents, who gave him injections and performed blood-glucose monitoring. When Robin entered junior high school 1 year ago, his parents gave him total responsibility for his diabetes management. Since then, he has been hospitalized five times for treatment of diabetic ketoacidosis (DKA). None of these episodes was precipitated by illness.

Questions 1 to 4 refer to this situation.

1 What is the most likely cause of Robin's recurrent DKA?

A. Onset of puberty, causing insulin resistance
B. Overeating and eating of concentrated sweets
C. Erratic insulin administration
D. Hypoglycemia with rebound hyperglycemia

2 Robin's parents do not want to believe that Robin is missing insulin injections. They have talked to him about future diabetic complications, and they feel that he understands the importance of good glucose control. Which statement by the nurse would help Robin's parents understand his developmental stage as it relates to his ability to manage his diabetes?

A. "Young adolescents have difficulty conceptualizing the distant future. They cannot comprehend reaching an age at which diabetes complications can develop"
B. "Young adolescents are too immature to be responsible for their own diabetes care. You should not have transferred so much responsibility to him at such a young age"
C. "Robin seems to be immature for his age. You should insist that he take on more chores at home in addition to managing his diabetes"
D. "Perhaps grounding Robin and eliminating his extracurricular activities will make him comply with his diabetes self-management"

3 Robin tells the nurse that he feels overwhelmed by assuming total responsibility for his diabetes care. He also says that he does not mind being in the hospital. Which associated benefits might Robin be achieving from his recurrent hospitalizations?

A. Increased attention from his parents, who are busy with their careers and younger children at home
B. Avoidance of stressful situations and difficult academic subjects at school
C. Reassurance that the adults in his life (parents, physicians, and nurses) are still available for him
D. All of the above

4 Robin asks the nurse to help him negotiate a contract with his parents regarding his diabetes care tasks. Considering Robin's developmental stage and his parents' busy schedules, which option is most feasible?

A. Robin's parents will take over all injections and blood testing
B. Robin will do the blood testing, his mother will give him a morning injection, and his father will give him an evening injection
C. Robin's insulin regimen will be reduced to one injection a day
D. None of the above

SITUATION

Chloe Reeves, age 18 months, has been ill for 4 days with lethargy, decreased appetite, and intermittent vomiting. For 2 weeks before this illness, she had been thirsty, often waking at night for a bottle. Mrs. Reeves tells the nurse that Chloe has had an increased number of wet diapers in the past 2 weeks along with a persistent diaper rash. She brought Chloe to the emergency department (ED) after the child suddenly lost interest in playing, began breathing heavily, and developed sunken eyes. Initial laboratory values include blood glucose level, 392 mg/dl; serum ketone levels, positive; serum potassium level, 4.2 mEq/liter; serum sodium, 131 mEq/liter; arterial pH, 6.96; and serum bicarbonate level, 15 mEq/liter. The physician diagnoses DKA.

Questions 5 to 8 refer to this situation.

5 Which signs and symptoms commonly manifest when a child develops diabetes mellitus?

A. Polyuria, polydipsia, and weight loss
B. Abnormally low urine specific gravity
C. Nocturnal enuresis or nocturia
D. Both A and C

6 Treatment goals for Chloe include:

A. Gradually reducing blood glucose levels (100 mg/dl/hour)
B. Clearing serum ketones by 24 hours
C. Restoring normal blood pH values
D. All of the above

7 When Chloe entered the ED, her blood pressure was 92/58 mm Hg and her pulse was 100 beats/minute; she was alert and able to recognize her parents. Four hours after receiving an infusion of I.V. fluids, her blood pressure is 120/82, her pulse rate is 78, and she cannot be aroused. Which treatment complication is Chloe most likely experiencing?

A. Hypokalemia
B. Cerebral edema
C. Hypoglycemia
D. Hyperglycemia

8 Nursing care of Chloe should include:

A. Monitoring urine specific gravity hourly
B. Catheterizing the child, even if she is alert enough to void at regular intervals
C. Administering insulin and I.V. fluids and observing for signs and symptoms of complications
D. Limiting environmental stimuli and parental visits

SITUATION

William Boyer, age 6 weeks, is brought to a rural clinic for his first well-baby checkup. The infant has mottled extremities, a large umbilical hernia, a large protruding tongue, and a hoarse cry. His parents report that he is constipated, sleeps for long periods, and lacks interest in feeding. He was born at home and has not received standard neonatal screening tests, such as those for phenylketonuria, hypothyroidism, and sickle cell disease.

Questions 9 to 12 refer to this situation.

9 Which congenital disorder is likely to be discovered when William is tested?

A. Phenylketonuria
B. Hypothyroidism
C. Sickle cell disease
D. Muscular dystrophy

10 What is the most important reason for immediately initiating thyroxine treatment for William?

A. To promote normal bowel motility
B. To promote normal neurologic development
C. To promote interest in feeding
D. To promote linear growth

11 To determine William's response to thyroxine treatment, the nurse should regularly evaluate his:

A. Visual development
B. Height and weight
C. Blood iodine levels
D. Blood iron-binding capacity levels

12 At a follow-up visit, Mr. and Mrs. Boyer report that they have difficulty remembering to give William his thyroxine every day. How should the nurse respond?

A. Review the importance of daily thyroxine therapy
B. Suggest the use of a small medication container with separate compartments for each day of the week
C. Discuss the family's daily routine and determine the best time of day for medication administration
D. All of the above

SITUATION

Baby Yeager is admitted to the neonatal nursery shortly after delivery. The obstetrician informs the parents that the sex of the neonate is ambiguous. Although otherwise healthy, the neonate has what appears to be an enlarged clitoris or a small phallus and scrotal tissue with no palpable testicles. The origin of the urine stream is not certain. The obstetrician tells Mr. and Mrs. Yeager that he thinks the child is probably a girl with an endocrine disorder. The admitting diagnosis is congenital adrenogenital hyperplasia.

Questions 13 and 14 refer to this situation.

13 What is the karyotype (chromosomal pattern) of an infant girl with congenital adrenogenital hyperplasia?

  A. Normal XX female karyotype
  B. Normal XY male karyotype
  C. XO (missing one X chromosome) karyotype
  D. None of the above

14 Mr. Yeager asks the nurse to explain congenital adrenogenital hyperplasia. The nurse correctly responds that:

  A. The neonate has an excessive amount of male hormones
  B. The neonate should be raised as a male
  C. The neonate was unable to produce cortisone in utero
  D. The neonate's sex may be undetermined for a while

SITUATION

Timmy Webb, age 3, is admitted to the pediatric unit with an elevated blood glucose level. His urine tests positive for sugar and ketones. Mrs. Webb reports that Timmy has been drinking and urinating more recently. His appetite also has increased, yet he has not gained weight. Timmy is diagnosed with type I diabetes mellitus.

Questions 15 to 17 refer to this situation.

15 The nurse can best determine Timmy's metabolic needs by:

  A. Measuring his blood glucose level after each meal, at bedtime, and during the night
  B. Carefully monitoring for glucose and ketones in urine and signs of hyperglycemia after each meal and at bedtime
  C. Checking his blood glucose level and monitoring for signs of hypoglycemia before each meal, at bedtime, and during the night
  D. Testing for glycosuria and ketonuria after each voiding

16 Which nursing action is necessary when administering combination doses of rapid- and intermediate-acting insulins?

A. Administering the insulin intramuscularly, paying careful attention to site rotation
B. Waiting at least 5 minutes before administering rapid- and intermediate-acting insulin that are drawn up in the same syringe
C. Administering intermediate-acting insulin immediately after meals to control blood glucose elevations
D. Administering the insulin ½ hour before breakfast and dinner

17 When teaching Timmy and his parents to manage diabetes, the nurse must:

A. Stress the importance of adhering to a rigid dietary regimen
B. Remind Timmy's parents to restrict his physical activity
C. Encourage Timmy and his parents to lead a normal life-style
D. Inform Timmy's parents to adjust his insulin dosage and diet based on his behavior

---

SITUATION

Steven, age 10, has had type I diabetes mellitus for 3 years. Recently, he developed an infection, a temperature of 102.8° F (39.3° C), and blood glucose levels ranging from 200 to 400 mg/dl.

Questions 18 and 19 refer to this situation.

18 Based on his blood glucose readings, Steven may require insulin every 4 hours. Which form of insulin is appropriate for this regimen?

A. NPH
B. Human
C. Regular
D. Lente

19 The nurse tests Steven's urine every 4 hours. When performing a urine test, the nurse must:

A. Use a sterile container for specimen collection
B. Time the test exactly, as stated in the directions
C. Verify the color changes with another nurse
D. All of the above

Answer sheet

	A	B	C	D
1	○	○	○	○
2	○	○	○	○
3	○	○	○	○
4	○	○	○	○
5	○	○	○	○
6	○	○	○	○
7	○	○	○	○
8	○	○	○	○
9	○	○	○	○
10	○	○	○	○
11	○	○	○	○
12	○	○	○	○
13	○	○	○	○
14	○	○	○	○
15	○	○	○	○
16	○	○	○	○
17	○	○	○	○
18	○	○	○	○
19	○	○	○	○

Answers and rationales

1 Correct answer—**C**

Diabetic ketoacidosis (DKA) is a state of extreme or complete insulin deficiency. Erratic insulin administration appears to be the
cause of Robin's recurrent DKA. Puberty and dietary noncompli-
ance could be minor contributing factors, but these were not men-
tioned in the situation. Hypoglycemia with rebound hyperglycemia (known as the Somogyi effect) can contribute to DKA in
persons receiving high doses of insulin. Because DKA was not a
problem before Robin's self-management of his diabetes, the
Somogyi effect is unlikely to be the cause of his recurrent episodes of DKA.

2 Correct answer—**A**

Young adolescents have difficulty conceptualizing the distant future and tend to believe that they are invulnerable to illness and
disease. Thus children of this age-group commonly experiment
with diabetes self-management. Most adolescents are developmentally capable of assuming responsibility for their diabetes care.
Children as young as age 9 or 10 can be taught to administer insulin; young school-age children (ages 6 to 8) can assume some responsibility for testing procedures. Telling the parents that they
were wrong to transfer care to their son is inappropriate and judgmental. Having Robin take on more chores in addition to his diabetes management may be too overwhelming and exacerbate the
problem. Diabetes care requires life-style changes that tend to
make an adolescent feel different from his peers at a time when
conformity and peer interaction are most important. Restricting
peer interaction and focusing on his illness would magnify
Robin's feelings of isolation; adolescents commonly rebel against
this parental approach.

3 Correct answer—**D**

Hospitalization may provide an adolescent with associated psychosocial benefits, such as increased attention from parents and
significant others. Hospitalization also provides a legitimate
means of avoiding school and may be used consciously or subcon-
sciously to escape stressful situations. Although adolescents are in
the process of establishing independence, they need reassurance
that the adults in their life are still available for them.

4 Correct answer—**B**

Because Robin is overwhelmed by his diabetes care tasks, the best solution is for him to maintain responsibility for blood testing while his parents manage the insulin injections. This approach balances Robin's need to assume self-care responsibilities with his need to be relieved from some aspects of diabetes care. His parents should not assume all the responsibility at a time when he should be learning self-management skills. Adolescents rarely achieve good glucose control with only one daily insulin injection. Most pediatric patients receive two daily injections, a regimen that is designed to approximate the body's normal insulin secretion pattern.

5 Correct answer—**D**

Polyuria, polydipsia, weight loss, and nocturia or nocturnal enuresis are caused by a lack of adequate insulin secretion. These symptoms commonly occur at the onset of diabetes in children. Polyuria, nocturia, or nocturnal enuresis are caused by hyperglycemia, which leads to osmotic diuresis. This diuresis causes dehydration, which leads to polydipsia. Weight loss occurs when body tissues break down to meet energy requirements. The presence of glucose in the urine is responsible for a high specific gravity.

6 Correct answer—**D**

DKA is a life-threatening condition; treatment aims to reverse the ketoacidosis. Therefore, the treatment goals for a child with DKA include gradual reduction in glucose levels, clearance of serum ketones, and restoration of normal blood pH values.

7 Correct answer—**B**

Altered neurologic status, decreased pulse rate, and increased blood pressure are signs of cerebral edema, a complication resulting from rehydration with solutions that are hypotonic to the patient's osmolality. Signs and symptoms of hypokalemia include hypotension, bradycardia or tachycardia, apathy, and drowsiness. Hypoglycemia is characterized by tachycardia and difficulty concentrating; hyperglycemia, by confusion and a slow, weak pulse.

8 Correct answer—**C**

A child with DKA has a severe insulin deficiency; therefore, the nurse must administer insulin and I.V. fluids. Monitoring urine specific gravity is inappropriate because this value is always elevated in a patient with glucosuria. A person with DKA has extremely high blood glucose levels; therefore, glucosuria is always present because the excess glucose is excreted in the urine. The nurse should not catheterize the child because this may lead to urinary tract infections in a diabetic patient; glucose in the urine provides an ideal environment for proliferation of microorganisms. Parental visits should not be restricted; an 18-month-old child can become extremely anxious when away from her parents; separation from parents may be the greatest stress imposed on such a hospitalized child.

9 Correct answer—**B**

Congenital hypothyroidism—a condition that causes insufficient secretion of thyroid hormones—can be intrinsic or related to exogenous intrauterine factors. Diagnosis of this disorder is made during infancy; the incidence is 1 in 4,000 births. Symptoms of congenital hypothyroidism include mottled and dry skin, umbilical hernia, constipation, large tongue, hoarse cry, excessive sleepiness, and lack of interest in feeding. Decreased metabolic rate and temperature regulation problems commonly result in intolerance to cold. The symptoms of juvenile hypothyoidism (hypothyroidism diagnosed after infancy) depend on the degree of thyroid dysfunction and the age of onset.

Phenylketonuria is a genetic disorder in which a person lacks the enzyme necessary for metabolizing phenylalanine. Buildup of phenylalanine affects the central nervous system (CNS) and results in mental retardation. Symptoms include failure to thrive, frequent vomiting, irritability, and hyperactive and peculiar behaviors. Sickle cell disease is a genetic disorder involving abnormally shaped hemoglobin. These distorted red blood cells cause clumping and obstruction. Symptoms include episodes of pain and signs of ischemia in the spleen, liver, and kidneys. Muscular dystrophy, a genetic disorder, is characterized by progressive weakness and muscle wasting.

10 Correct answer—**B**

The most important reason for initiating thyroxine therapy is to promote neurologic development. Thyroxine regulates the metabolic rate of all cells and promotes tissue differentiation. During the first 2 to 3 years, when significant CNS growth occurs, insufficient thryoxine can impair neurologic development. Intellectual capacity is severely affected by a delay in thyroxine replacement. Normalizing the infant's thyroxine levels also promotes bowel motility, increases appetite, and fosters normal growth. However, these effects are not the primary reason for starting thyroxine therapy.

11 Correct answer—**B**

Careful assessment of an infant's physical and cognitive development is important. Most infants with congenital hypothyroidism are evaluated at 3-month intervals until age 2; brain growth is complete by ages 2 to 3. Thyroid levels must be monitored regularly to prevent overdosage of thyroxine. Visual disturbances are not characteristic of hypothyroidism. Measurements of blood iodine levels are helpful for diagnosing hypothyroidism but not for determining a response to treatment. Iron-binding capacity measurements are helpful in diagnosing anemia, not hypothyroidism.

12 Correct answer—**D**

The parents must understand that inadequate therapy can adversely affect their child's neurologic development and intelligence. Thus, reviewing the importance of daily thyroxine therapy should improve compliance. Using medication containers with separate compartments may help the parents remember to administer the medication. Minimizing disruptions in daily routine and pairing medication administration with a daily activity also may increase compliance with the therapeutic regimen. A child who receives thyroxine in the evening may have difficulty sleeping. However, if evening is the most convenient time to administer the medication, establishing this timetable helps to ensure regular administration.

13 Correct answer—**A**

A girl with congenital adrenogenital hyperplasia has a normal female chromosomal pattern; however, her external genitalia have been virilized because of excessive testosterone production by the adrenal cortex. Surgical exploration typically reveals a normal uterus, ovaries, and vagina.

14 Correct answer—C

The nurse should explain that, while in utero, the neonate was unable to produce cortisone; as a result, the glands responsible for making cortisone produced too much testosterone, which enlarged the clitoris and fused the labia. Explaining that the neonate has an excessive amount of male hormones suggests that this imbalance is permanent, which is not the case. Before the 20th century, many girls with congenital adrenogenital hyperplasia were mistakenly raised as boys. Today, physicians can use ultrasound to quickly determine the child's sex by visualizing the internal structures for the presence of female sex organs. Chromosomal analysis is performed to determine the neonate's genotype, but the results of this test are not immediately available. Congenital adrenogenital hyperplasia is treated with cortisol.

15 Correct answer—C

The blood glucose level should be elevated after meals; therefore, the nurse should measure the levels by glucometer or glucose test strips while the child is in a fasting state (before each meal, at bedtime, and, if necessary, during the night) to determine if they are within normal limits. Urine tests for glucose and acetone are also done before meals. This parameter is less accurate, however, because urine does not reflect the current blood glucose level.

16 Correct answer—D

Diabetes in children usually is managed with two daily injections consisting of a combined dose of rapid- and intermediate-acting insulins. The insulin is administered ½ hour before breakfast and dinner. Regular (rapid-acting) insulin counteracts the immediate rise in blood glucose after a meal. Intermediate-acting insulin maintains normal values as the body continues to metabolize the food. Both types of insulin are drawn up in the same syringe so that they can be given as one injection. To prevent the rapid-acting insulin from combining with the intermediate-acting insulin (which could produce a longer-acting form), the insulin should be injected immediately or within 5 minutes after being drawn up into the syringe. Insulin is administered subcutaneously, not intramuscularly.

17 Correct answer—C

The nurse should encourage the parents of a diabetic child to think of the child as a person with specific health needs that can be adapted to a normal life-style. Some flexibility in menu planning is allowed and encouraged because rigidity can lead to future non-compliance. Physical activity is recommended, although the effects of exercise on insulin requirements must be considered. Insulin and dietary adjustments should be based on blood glucose values, not the child's behavior. Behavior is a poor gauge of glucose fluctuations. Both hypoglycemia and hyperglycemia initially manifest as behavior changes; distinguishing between the two is difficult.

18 Correct answer—C

Regular insulin is given every 4 hours because of its short duration of action. Its onset occurs within ½ hour; its peak effect, within 2 to 3 hours. It has a duration of action of 4 to 5 hours. NPH is an intermediate-acting insulin, with an onset of 1 to 2 hours, peak effect at 8 to 13 hours, and duration of action of up to 24 hours. Lente is a long-acting insulin preparation, with an onset of 4 to 8 hours, peak effect at 14 to 20 hours, and duration of action of more than 36 hours. Human insulin describes the source of the insulin, not its duration of action. This type of insulin is less allergenic than the animal varieties and may be appropriate for persons who are sensitive or resistant to other types of insulin.

19 Correct answer—B

Urine testing strips change color and deteriorate over time. Therefore, the nurse must follow the directions exactly to ensure a correct reading. The amount of glucose in the urine is not affected by the type of container used. If the nurse has difficulty verifying the color changes, checking with another nurse may help; however, this usually is not necessary.

CHAPTER 12

Respiratory Disorders

Questions

1 Which respiratory rate is considered normal for a 5-year-old child?

   A. 15 to 20 breaths/minute
   B. 20 to 25 breaths/minute
   C. 25 to 30 breaths/minute
   D. 30 to 35 breaths/minute

2 Respiratory function for gas exchange consists of ventilation, perfusion, and:

   A. Diffusion
   B. Osmosis
   C. Transport
   D. Inhalation

3 Which muscle or muscle group is principally involved in respiration?

   A. Intercostal muscles
   B. Diaphragm
   C. Vastus lateralis
   D. Rectus femoris

4 Which information is most important when assessing a child with a suspected respiratory tract infection?

   A. Hydration status
   B. School activity
   C. Immunization reports
   D. Surrounding vegetation

5 All of the following observations indicate respiratory distress in an infant *except:*

   A. Substernal retractions
   B. Rapid deep breathing
   C. Grunting
   D. Noisy breathing

6 Chest physiotherapy includes postural drainage, percussion, and:

A. Perfusion
B. Diffusion
C. Suction
D. Vibration

7 Clinical manifestations of pneumonia in a child include:

A. Paroxysmal, dry, harsh cough
B. Dyspnea and deep respirations
C. Marked intercostal retractions
D. Fever and tachypnea

8 Therapy for childhood pneumonia primarily depends on:

A. Nose and throat cultures
B. Clinical symptoms and history
C. Sputum cultures
D. Chest X-ray

SITUATION

Derick Peterson, age 3 months, was treated for respiratory distress syndrome at birth. Initially, he required continuous positive airway pressure (CPAP), followed by 2 weeks of 100% oxygen and mechanical ventilation. Attempts to discontinue his respiratory support were unsuccessful. He still requires 40% oxygen, and X-rays show chronic changes with hyperinflation. Derick's fluid intake is restricted, and he is receiving hypertonic formula. He has not gained weight over the past month. The pediatrician diagnoses bronchopulmonary dysplasia (BPD).

Questions 9 to 12 refer to this situation.

9 Precipitating factors related to BPD include:

A. Polycythemia and tachypnea
B. CPAP and oropharangeal suctioning
C. Mechanical ventilation and high oxygen concentrations
D. Retained fetal lung fluid and tachypnea

10 Which outcome indicates effective management of an infant with BPD?

A. The infant meets developmental milestones in a timely manner
B. The infant has improved ventilation when positioned on his abdomen
C. The infant takes in large amounts of formula with each feeding
D. The infant shows improved pulmonary function as he gains weight

11 When teaching Mr. and Mrs. Peterson about home apnea monitoring, the nurse must stress that Derick should be connected to the monitor:

A. Continuously, even during his bath
B. Continuously, except when being held by a caregiver competent in assessment and resuscitation
C. Only when the caregiver is not in the room
D. Only when sleeping at night, when he is at highest risk for sudden infant death syndrome

12 What is the expected prognosis for an infant with BPD?

A. Poor because of his susceptibility to pneumonia and respiratory infections
B. Fair because he will be oxygen-dependent for his entire life
C. Fair because he probably will outgrow BPD but will develop asthma
D. Good because he probably will outgrow BPD if the disease is mild

SITUATION

Sonja Mathis, age 13 months, has a history of repeated upper respiratory tract infections and poor weight gain. She was admitted to the hospital with pneumonia 3 days ago; today she is diagnosed with cystic fibrosis.

Questions 13 to 15 refer to this situation.

13 Nursing care for Sonja should involve all of the following *except:*

A. Preventing infection
B. Maintaining nutritional needs
C. Assisting with oxygenation
D. Preventing disease transmission

14 Which nursing intervention should the nurse include in Sonja's care plan?

A. Monitoring Sonja's blood glucose level four time a day
B. Performing postural drainage with percussion three times a day
C. Accompanying Sonja to physical therapy daily
D. Placing Sonja in protective (reverse) isolation

15 The physician prescribes pancrelipase (Pancrease) for Sonja to:

A. Soften stools and prevent constipation
B. Prevent an allergic reaction to milk
C. Supply needed enzymes to digest food
D. Prevent upper respiratory tract infections

SITUATION

Karen Shriver, age 18 months, is admitted to the pediatric unit with a diagnosis of bronchiolitis. She has an elevated temperature, is pale, and looks tired. She also appears to be mildly dyspneic. The physician prescribes administration of 30% oxygen with mist.

Questions 16 to 19 refer to this situation.

16 The admitting nurse should ensure that Karen's room includes:

A. A tracheostomy set
B. A croup tent
C. A sign indicating the need for respiratory isolation
D. A portable chest X-ray machine

17 While Karen is receiving humidified oxygen, the nurse must be concerned with:

A. Keeping the mist level low enough so that her pajamas and bedding remain dry
B. Caring for the areas of skin under the nasal cannula
C. Preventing oxygen toxicity in the tent
D. Keeping the edges of the tent tucked under the blankets

18 Karen has been refusing fluids for the past 24 hours. Besides administering I.V. fluids as prescribed by the physician, how can the nurse ensure oral rehydration?

A. Ask Karen's mother to bring in some of Karen's favorite beverages
B. Place a bottle of apple juice in Karen's bed
C. Hold Karen and spoon-feed her sips of fluid
D. Wake Karen and give her fluids every hour

19 By the third day of hospitalization, Karen is allowed to remain outside the tent for brief periods. After 20 minutes of playing quietly on her mother's lap, her heart rate is 130 beats/minute, respirations are 32 breaths/minute, and her nares are flared. The nurse determines that Karen requires:

A. Immediate placent in the oxygen tent
B. Prompt attention from her physician
C. A nap
D. A bottle or another comfort measure

SITUATION

Shannon O'Connor, age 2¹/₂, is admitted to the pediatric unit with a diagnosis of laryngotracheobronchitis (croup). The physician prescribes an aerosol tent with cool mist and an infusion of dextrose 5% in 0.45% (half-normal) saline solution. Shannon's vital signs are: heart rate, 130 beats/minute; respiratory rate, 30 breaths/minute; and rectal temperature, 102° F (38.8° C).

Questions 20 to 22 refer to this situation.

20 The physician prescribes a croup tent with mist because it:

A. Provides a steady supply of oxygen, thereby easing respiratory effort
B. Helps to liquefy secretions, making expectoration easier
C. Provides an isolated environment for this infectious condition
D. Helps to suppress coughing episodes

21 In addition to feeling sick, Shannon seems to be extremely frightened. She continually tries to climb out of her tent and bed. Which nursing measure will help to lessen Shannon's anxiety?

A. Allowing another child with croup to play with Shannon in her tent
B. Allowing Mrs. O'Connor to enter the tent and stand next to Shannon's bed
C. Placing books and stuffed animals in Shannon's tent
D. Placing a battery-powered toy in Shannon's tent

22 Mrs. O'Connor asks the nurse to explain croup. After hearing about its causes, signs, symptoms, and prognosis, Mrs. O'Connor remarks, "Well, I'm certainly glad that my daughter won't be going through this again." The nurse interprets this reply as:

A. A need for more instruction about possible recurrences
B. A demonstration of the mother's full understanding of her child's respiratory health
C. An accurate account of the disease
D. An indication of the mother's realization that croup is rare after age 2

SITUATION

Brenda Martz, age 3, is brought to the pediatric clinic by her mother, who reports that Brenda has a sore throat and fever and will not eat or drink. The physician diagnoses epiglottitis.

Questions 23 and 24 refer to this situation.

23 Which symptoms are associated with epiglottitis?

A. Dyspnea, restlessness, hoarseness, and moaning
B. Leaning forward, anxiety, drooling, and a muffled voice
C. Crouching, leaning with hands stretched out in back, and extended neck
D. Ruddy complexion, distended neck veins, and knee-chest position

24 The nurse's first action when caring for Brenda should be to:

A. Obtain a tracheostomy set and notify the physician
B. Begin respiratory precautions immediately
C. Obtain I.V. and oxygen equipment
D. Obtain a cardiac monitor and an emergency equipment cart

SITUATION

Megan Lowell, age 6, has had recurrent tonsillitis, adenitis, and high fevers during the past year. She also drools excessively, breathes through her mouth, speaks in a nasal tone, and has difficulty hearing. Her tonsils are enlarged and inflamed. She is admitted to the pediatric unit for a tonsillectomy and adenoidectomy. The nurse notes that Megan appears frightened.

Questions 25 to 29 refer to this situation.

25 Preoperatively, the nurse should pay particular attention to Megan's:

A. Urine specific gravity
B. Pulse and respiratory rates
C. Bleeding and clotting times
D. Blood pressure taken in the supine and sitting positions

26 Megan's surgery is postponed for a few days. What is the most likely reason for the delay?

A. Megan has a loose tooth
B. Megan's tonsils are infected
C. Megan's behavior has regressed since her admission
D. Megan is fearful, even after preoperative explanations

27 Megan's preoperative anxiety may be alleviated by:

A. Explaining that she will not feel any pain after her injection
B. Using a doll to explain the procedure
C. Talking about her next birthday and the gifts she wants
D. Telling her that her parents will be with her at all times

28 After Megan is taken to the operating room, the nurse prepares her room for her return. Which equipment is needed at the bedside postoperatively?

A. Otoscope, oral thermometer, and suction machine
B. Flashlight, sphygmomanometer, and shock blocks
C. Tongue blade, flashlight, and suction machine
D. Oxygen setup, mist tent, and tongue blade

29 The nurse should suspect postoperative bleeding if Megan displays which symptoms?

A. Pain, anxiety, and dark brown blood in emesis and nose
B. Restlessness, frequent swallowing, throat clearing, and increased pulse rate
C. Increased pulse rate and respirations and a temperature of 103° F (39.4° C)
D. Decreased pulse rate, throat clearing, and pain

SITUATION

Arlene Hicks, age 2, is admitted to the pediatric unit after being treated in the emergency department (ED) for status asthmaticus. Upon arrival on the unit, Arlene is receiving an I.V. theophylline drip and a maintenance solution of dextrose 5% in a 0.2% saline solution.

Questions 30 to 33 refer to this situation.

30 Status asthmaticus is a form of asthma that is:

A. Always fatal
B. Controlled by epinephrine injections
C. Contagious
D. Difficult to control

31 A recent nursing graduate asks the primary nurse why Arlene is receiving theophylline I.V. She is confused because Arlene received an injection of epinephrine 2 hours ago in the ED, and both drugs are bronchodilators. The nurse correctly responds by saying:

A. "Epinephrine causes nausea and vomiting, and theophylline does not"
B. "Epinephrine is extremely potent, but its effects have worn off long ago"
C. "Epinephrine is a corticosteroid, and it's best to discontinue such drugs as soon as possible"
D. "Theophylline has no cardiotoxic effects"

32 Arlene is being discharged with a prescription for oral theophylline (Slo-Bid). Mrs. Hicks asks the nurse if she should purchase a portable inhalation device that administers over-the-counter (OTC) drugs in measured doses to use in an acute asthma attack. The nurse's best response would be:

A. "Talk to the physician. Sometimes OTC drugs are incompatible with prescription drugs"
B. "Inhalation devices are never recommended for children with asthma because they can become contaminated with bacteria"
C. "If your daughter starts using an inhalation device now, she will be physically dependent on it by the time she is 6 years old"
D. "Any OTC medication intended for use by patients with bronchial asthma is fine"

33 In preparing Arlene for discharge, the nurse should be primarily concerned with:

A. Arranging a follow-up appointment at the asthma clinic
B. Discussing strategies to rid the home of known allergens
C. Instructing Arlene's parents to restrict her activity
D. Teaching Arlene's parents about postural drainage

SITUATION

John Davies was just delivered vaginally at 32 weeks' gestation. His Apgar scores are 7 and 9. On admission to the neonatal nursery, he has a respiratory rate of 72 breaths/minute, moderate substernal retractions, nasal flaring, and expiratory grunting. The physician diagnoses respiratory distress syndrome (RDS).

Questions 34 and 35 refer to this situation.

34 Which sign is most characteristic of RDS?

A. Substernal retractions
B. Slight nasal flaring
C. Tachypnea
D. Audible expiratory grunting

35 Which intervention is the nurse's priority when John exhibits signs and symptoms of RDS?

A. Identifying his risk for hypoglycemia
B. Observing him closely for signs of increasing respiratory effort
C. Assessing for hypoxia and implementing measures to relieve it
D. Minimizing environmental stimulation

Answer sheet

	A B C D		A B C D
1	○○○○	**31**	○○○○
2	○○○○	**32**	○○○○
3	○○○○	**33**	○○○○
4	○○○○	**34**	○○○○
5	○○○○	**35**	○○○○
6	○○○○		
7	○○○○		
8	○○○○		
9	○○○○		
10	○○○○		
11	○○○○		
12	○○○○		
13	○○○○		
14	○○○○		
15	○○○○		
16	○○○○		
17	○○○○		
18	○○○○		
19	○○○○		
20	○○○○		
21	○○○○		
22	○○○○		
23	○○○○		
24	○○○○		
25	○○○○		
26	○○○○		
27	○○○○		
28	○○○○		
29	○○○○		
30	○○○○		

Answers and rationales

1 Correct answer—**B**

The respiratory rate for a healthy 5-year-old child is 20 to 25 breaths/minute. A rate of 40 to 60 breaths/minute is normal for a neonate, an obligatory nose breather. As the child grows, his respiratory rate decreases. An adult has a respiratory rate of 15 to 20 breaths/minute.

2 Correct answer—**A**

Ventilation, diffusion, and perfusion are the components of respiratory function for gas exchange. Ventilation is the movement of air into and out of the lungs. During inspiration, atmospheric gases move into the lungs with oxygenated air. During expiration, carbon dioxide is removed from the lungs. Perfusion is a process whereby oxygen is transported from pulmonary capillaries to body tissues via red blood cells and plasma. Diffusion allows for the transfer of inhaled gas across the alveolocapillary membrane to the capillaries of the lung. This passive process also allows oxygen to reach the erythrocytes in the circulatory system. Osmosis is the passage of a solvent (usually water) through a membrane from an area of lower concentration of solute (a substance dissolved in solution) to an area of higher concentration in an attempt to equalize the concentration of the two solutions. Inhalation is the act of drawing air into the lungs.

3 Correct answer—**B**

The diaphragm is the principal muscle used in respiration. Contraction of the diaphragm lengthens the chest cavity and increases the volume of this area during inspiration. Infants and young children rely primarily on diaphragmatic breathing. The intercostal muscles in children are not well developed. In adults, these muscles raise the ribs during inspiration, resulting in increased chest cavity volume. The vastus lateralis and rectus femoris are muscles found in the thighs; they have no bearing on respiration.

4 Correct answer—**C**

When assessing a child with a suspected respiratory tract infection, the nurse must note any contributing factors, including the child's nutritional status, living conditions and sanitation, exposure to illness or disease, delays in immunizations, travel, and results of tuberculin tests. These factors provide data about the possible causes of the infection. Subsequent interventions and treatment, such as respiratory isolation and antibiotic therapy, are based on the cause of the infection. The nurse also must assess the child's hydration status because dehydration is associated with respiratory tract infections; however, this information is not as important as identifying the cause of infection. An assessment of surrounding vegetation is pertinent when allergic rhinitis or asthma is suspected. School activity is irrelevant in this situation.

5 Correct answer—B

An infant in respiratory distress typically exhibits rapid, shallow respirations, circumoral cyanosis, nasal flaring, and intercostal and substernal retractions, grunting, and noisy breathing. Rapid deep breathing is characteristic of metabolic acidosis.

6 Correct answer—D

Chest physiotherapy (CPT) consists of postural drainage, percussion, and vibration. These three interventions stimulate productive coughing to clear the airways and remove secretions. Postural drainage, which is performed in 20- to 30-minute sessions, facilitates removal of secretions through the use of gravity. The position used depends on the lung segment to be drained. Percussion (vigorous clapping of the chest wall with a cupped hand) is performed during postural drainage to loosen secretions; it is never performed over bare skin or near the sternum, spine, stomach, or kidneys. Vibration—delivery of a rapid vibratory impulse with the hand over a lung segment—is performed during the expiratory phase of respiration. Perfusion and diffusion are elements of gas exchange. Suction—mechanical removal of mucus and secretions from the respiratory tract—is not a part of CPT.

7 Correct answer—D

Clinical manifestations of pneumonia in a child include fatigue, irritability, anxiety, dyspnea, shallow respirations, productive cough, fever, and tachypnea. Mild to moderate intercostal retractions also may be present. A young child with pneumonia also may have vomiting and anorexia.

8 Correct answer—B

Because the infectious organism is typically difficult to isolate, therapy for childhood pneumonia is based on the child's clinical symptoms and medical history. Clinical symptoms can help to distinguish the type of pneumonia (viral, bacterial, mycoplasm, or aspiration). The medical history can provide information about the cause (for example, a child with staphylococcal pneumonia typically has a history of recent staphylococcal skin infection). Nose and throat cultures may or may not help to identify the cause of the infection. Although a sputum culture can help in identifying the causative organism, obtaining a sputum specimen from a child is particularly difficult because it necessitates expectoration. Chest X-rays may be used to confirm pleural effusion or lung consolidation, which can aid in diagnosis.

9 Correct answer—C

Bronchopulmonary dysplasia (BPD) is a persistent form of respiratory distress that usually follows severe respiratory distress syndrome. Although the etiology of BPD is unknown, precipitating factors include oxygen toxicity, mechanical injury, chronic inflammation, and excessive fluid and sodium intake. BPD in infants is similar to adult respiratory distress syndrome. A combination of high concentrations of oxygen and high-pressure settings on a mechanical ventilator damage the airways and create a pulmonary hemorrhage, which leads to fibrosis. Chronic hypoxia, decreased pulmonary perfusion, and pulmonary hypertension with resultant cor pulmonale follow. Polycythemia and tachypnea are symptoms that indicate impaired oxygenation; they are not responsible for BPD. Neither oropharyngeal suctioning nor retained fetal lung fluid is a precipitating factor in BPD.

10 Correct answer—D

Adequate nutritional management is critical in an infant with BPD because malnutrition delays cell growth and the development of new alveoli. Proper nutrition and oxygenation help to improve pulmonary function in such a child. Expecting an infant with BPD to meet developmental milestones in a timely manner may be unrealistic becuase children with BPD commonly experience developmental delays from the lack of sensory stimulation caused by spending a significant amount of time in an oxygen tent. Because an infant uses his diaphragm and abdominal muscles for respiration, abdominal positioning would be detrimental to ventilation. Because the infant tires easily, large amounts of formula might compromise respiration; small, frequent feedings are better tolerated.

11 Correct answer—B

An infant with BPD is subject to apneic spells. Therefore, Derick should be connected to an apnea monitor at all times, unless he is being held by a caregiver who is competent in assessing his respiratory status and providing resuscitation. Apnea monitoring involves placement of electrodes on the infant's chest to detect respirations; an alarm sounds if respiration is delayed. An infant connected to a monitor should never be submerged in water because of the danger of electric shock. However, a light sponge bath may be given if the electrodes are protected from contact with water. An infant with BPD is not necessarily at increased risk for sudden infant death syndrome.

12 Correct answer—D

The long-term prognosis for an infant with BPD is generally good, but depends on the severity of the illness. Other conditions, diseases, congenital defects, treatment side effects, and quality of care after discharge affect the prognosis. Many infants with BPD outgrow their respiratory problems, are not oxygen-dependent, and lead normal lives. Although children who survive BPD may develop reactive airway problems, they do not usually develop asthma, pneumonia, or respiratory syncytial virus.

13 Correct answer—D

Cystic fibrosis is transmitted genetically by an autosomal recessive trait. Children with cystic fibrosis suffer frequent infections because the overproduction of mucus in their lungs provides an excellent medium for bacterial growth. However, the disease itself is not contagious. Maintaining adequate nutrition is important because cystic fibrosis impairs absorption of food and vitamins. Respiratory tract infections associated with this disorder necessitate assistance with oxygenation.

14 Correct answer—B

One of the most important therapies for improving respiratory function in a child with cystic fibrosis involves performing postural drainage with percussion several times a day. These procedures usually are preceded by inhalation therapy with bronchodilators. Inhalation therapy delivers moistened air to the respiratory tract, which loosens secretions and eases their removal. Frequent monitoring of the blood glucose level is appropriate for a child with diabetes, not cystic fibrosis. Physical therapy for a child with cystic fibrosis comprises postural drainage and breathing exercises, which are performed in the patient's room. Although Sonja is at risk for respiratory tract infections, reverse isolation is not necessary.

15 Correct answer—C

In a patient with cystic fibrosis, the pancreatic duct is blocked by mucus. Therefore, pancreatic enzymes (such as trypsin, amylase, and lipase), which aid in the digestion and absorption of fats and proteins, are absent or diminished. Pancrelipase (Pancrease) supplies the enzymes that are needed to digest food properly.

16 Correct answer—B

Bronchiolitis, a repiratory tract disease characterized by tenacious secretions, is generally treated by administration of humidified air. This involves delivering oxygen with mist via an enclosed tent that helps to thin the secretions. Tracheostomy is not indicated because the mucus obstructions occur in the bronchioles, which are below the trachea. A child with bronchiolitis does not require specific infection control precautions. Moving the child's bed away from others and practicing good hand-washing techniques are sufficient to prevent transmission to other children on the unit. Body fluid precautions are indicated in situations in which transmission of the pathogen occurs via blood or body fluids, such as with human immunodeficiency virus. Diagnosis of bronchiolitis is based on the child's medical history and physical examination findings, not on X-ray results.

17 Correct answer—D

Although an oxygen tent is bulky and an imprecise way to deliver oxygen, it is unobtrusive and better tolerated by a child than a mask or cannula. Because air can escape through the edges of the tent, the nurse should minimize oxygen loss by tucking the tent edges under the blankets. Condensation of the mist within the tent does not indicate that the mist level must be lowered. When oxygen is delivered via the tent method, a nasal cannula is unnecessary. Maintaining an oxygen level of greater than 40% in a tent is difficult because of air escape. Therefore, oxygen toxicity is not a primary concern.

18 Correct answer—**A**

An 18-month-old child probably has distinct likes and dislikes. Karen may be more inclined to drink liquids if her favorite beverages are on hand. A child who has been refusing fluids would not be motivated to pick up a bottle of juice; a child of Karen's age also is more likely to be drinking from a cup. Holding Karen and spoon-feeding her fluids necessitates removing her from the humidified, oxygenated environment that is part of her treatment. Waking Karen and giving her fluids every hour is inadvisable because rest is extremely important for a child with bronchiolitis. Rest minimizes the body's oxygen needs at a time when air exchange is compromised.

19 Correct answer—**A**

Karen's respiratory and heart rates indicate mild tachypnea and tachycardia. These vital sign deviations and the presence of nasal flaring signify insufficient oxygenation and the need for immediate oxygen-assisted breathing. Contacting the physician is unnecessary unless the patient's situation does not improve when she is returned to the tent. Lack of oxygen, not lack of sleep or comfort, is the cause of Karen's symptoms.

20 Correct answer—**B**

The mist in an aerosol (croup) tent provides fine droplets of humidified air that reach into affected areas to thin the patient's mucus. In this case, concentrated oxygen is not delivered; the air supply is of the same composition as the room air. The mist contained in the aerosol tent stimulates productive coughing, which helps to clear the secretions. An isolation environment or other specific infection control measures are unnecessary for patients with acute laryngotracheobronchitis.

21 Correct answer—**B**

At age 2½, Shannon's greatest fear is separation from her parents. Providing a way for her to be close to her mother while maintaining compliance with the medical regimen is part of the challenge of meeting Shannon's needs. Because croup may be caused by a viral or bacterial infection, cross-contamination could be a problem if Shannon is allowed tô play with another child. Books would not hold her interest for long, and a stuffed animal that is

placed in a mist tent will become moist and harbor bacteria. Only
toys that can be wiped off easily should be placed in the tent, with
the possible exception of one of the child's best-loved objects. If
oxygen is being delivered in the tent, a battery-powered toy could
be dangerous; the current passing through such a toy may cause
oxygen combustion.

22 Correct answer—A

Having a croup attack does not protect a child against subsequent
episodes. Therefore, the nurse should interpret Mrs. O'connor's
statement as a need for further instruction about the possible recurrences associated with this disorder. Croup is not rare after age 2;
however, most cases occur before age 3.

23 Correct answer—B

Leaning forward, anxiety, drooling, and a muffled voice are the
classic symptoms of epiglottitis. The child typically assumes a sitting, forward-leaning position, which minimizes the work of
breathing and facilitates the use of accessory muscles for respiration. The child's anxious expression may be related to her inability
to swallow and her progressive airway obstruction. Drooling and a
muffled voice also result from the inability to swallow caused by
swelling of the epiglottis. Hoarseness, moaning, distended neck
veins, and a ruddy complexion are not symptoms of epiglottitis. A
knee-chest position, crouching, and leaning with hands stretched
out in back impedes breathing and requires additional energy expenditure; a child with epiglottitis would not exhibit these signs.

24 Correct answer—A

Because of the speed with which complete obstruction can occur
in a patient with epiglottitis, airway equipment must be nearby
and a physician must be in attendance. Beginning respiratory precautions or obtaining I.V. and oxygen equipment ignore the fact
that this is an emergency. A cardiac monitor and an emergency
equipment cart are indicated for other disorders that are not associated with epiglottitis, such as cardiac or respiratory failure and arrhythmias.

25 Correct answer—C

Because the surgical site of a tonsillectomy and adenoidectomy is
highly vascular, bleeding and clotting times should be determined.

A complete blood count also is necessary to assess the patient's health. Urine specific gravity does not supply important data for a patient undergoing a tonsillectomy. Baseline blood pressure and pulse and respiratory rates should be obtained preoperatively, but they are not as critical as the patient's bleeding and clotting times.

26 Correct answer—B

Tonsillectomy and adenoidectomy are never performed if the tonsils and adenoids are infected because pathogenic organisms can spread into the bloodstream and cause septicemia. Performing surgery on infected tissue also increases the risk of bleeding. Loose teeth are not a problem because they are pulled, with the parent's permission, after anesthesia is given. Some degree of regressive behavior is common in hospitalized children and is not a reason to postpone surgery. Similarly, Megan's fear also is not a reason to delay the operation. Hospitalized school-age children commonly fear loss of control, bodily injury, pain, and to some extent, separation from parents.

27 Correct answer—B

A school-age child typically benefits from concrete explanations of surgical procedures. The nurse may use pictures and dolls to explain procedures in terms that the child can understand. Reassuring the child that only her tonsils and adenoids will be affected may decrease fears of bodily harm. The nurse should be honest when discussing the unpleasant aspects of surgery, such as postoperative pain. Talking about the child's birthday does not give Megan an opportunity to discuss her fears and concerns. Telling Megan that her parents will be with her at all times would be untrue; she may become upset on waking in the recovery room without her parents present. It also would decrease her trust in the nurse.

28 Correct answer—C

Postoperative hemorrhage is a possible complication of tonsillectomy and adenoidectomy. The nurse should observe the surgical site for signs of bleeding by carefully inserting a tongue blade into the child's mouth and visualizing the tonsillar area with a flashlight. Because edema or accumulated secretions can cause postoperative airway obstruction, a suction machine should be available at the patient's bedside. The equipment listed in the other options is not related to this procedure.

29 Correct answer—**B**

Because Megan may inadvertently swallow blood oozing from the surgical site postoperatively with no apparent sign of heavy bleeding, the nurse should assess for frequent swallowing and throat clearing as indications of postoperative bleeding. Other systemic indications of blood loss are restlessness, increased pulse rate (greater than 120 beats/minute), increased respiratory rate, and pallor.

30 Correct answer—**D**

Status asthmaticus is a form of asthma that does not respond to normal therapy, making it difficult to control. A physician typically diagnoses status asthmaticus when an individual does not respond to injections of epinephrine and inhaled beta-agonists. Treatment usually consists of infusions of aminophylline and steroids. The condition is fatal only if left untreated. Asthma is not contagious.

31 Correct answer—**B**

Epinephrine is a potent, rapid-acting bronchodilator with a short duration of action; it is not a corticosteroid. Nausea and vomiting are common side effects of both theophylline and epinephrine. Theophylline can produce cardiotoxic effects, including tachycardia and other life-threatening arrhythmias.

32 Correct answer—**A**

Over-the-counter inhaler preparations may contain multiple medications, which increases the risk of drug interactions. Therefore, parents should check with a physician or nurse before using such devices. Inhalers may become contaminated with bacteria and fungi, and parents should be instructed on the thorough cleaning of these devices. However, use of an inhalation device by children is not prohibited for this reason. No evidence suggests that children who use these devices become physically dependent on them.

33 Correct answer—**B**

The nurse's primary objective should be to prevent future asthma attacks. Once allergens have been identified, the nurse can recommend ways for the family to rid the home of the allergens or to minimize the child's exposure to them. Arlene's parents need not restrict her activity. Moderate exercise can be beneficial for children with asthma, and there is no indication that Arlene's attack was precipitated by exercise. The nurse can arrange for a follow-up clinic appointment and teach postural drainage if prescribed (not all asthmatic children require postural drainage). However, these actions would not prevent future asthma attacks.

34 Correct answer—D

An expiratory grunt, which is caused by partial closure of the glottis as the neonate attempts to maintain alveolar expansion, is characteristic of respiratory distress syndrome (RDS), or hyaline membrane disease. A neonate typically exhibits mild nasal flaring, retractions, and tachypnea after birth; however, these signs usually disappear spontaneously.

35 Correct answer—C

Hypoxia accentuates vascular spasm and pulmonary hypoperfusion and can cause capillary damage and alveolar necrosis. It also further impairs the production of surfactant. As surface tension continues to increase, atelectasis becomes more severe. Thus the nurse's priority is to assess for hypoxia and implement measures to relieve it. Interventions aimed at relieving hypoxia include the administration of supplemental oxygen and the use of assisted ventilation. Premature infants are commonly at risk for hypoglycemia, but identifying this risk is not a primary concern for this patient. Because John has demonstrated signs of RDS, observing for symptoms of increasing respiratory effort is insufficient—the nurse also must take steps to relieve the hypoxia. Although environmental stimulation and stress can contribute to hypoxia, measures to alleviate hypoxia would have a more profound effect on the neonate's condition than those to reduce stimulation or stress.

CHAPTER 13

Cardiovascular Disorders

Questions

1 Which of the following reduces the risk of endocarditis in a child with congenital heart disease?

A. Avoiding invasive procedures
B. Delaying routine immunizations
C. Maintaining continuous antibiotic prophylaxis
D. Maintaining good dental care

2 Cerebrovascular accident associated with congenital heart disease results mainly from:

A. Altered pulmonary blood flow
B. Cardiomegaly
C. Decreased exercise tolerance
D. Polycythemia

3 Blood pressure that varies among extremities is a common finding in children with:

A. Aortic stenosis
B. Coarctation of the aorta
C. Patent ductus arteriosus
D. Atrial septal defect

4 Which congenital cardiac anomaly is associated with tetralogy of Fallot (TOF)?

A. Origination of the aorta from the right ventricle and origination of the pulmonary artery from the left ventricle
B. A hole in the ventricular septum allowing communication between the ventricles
C. Pulmonary stenosis, right ventricular hypertrophy, ventricular septal defect, and dextroposition of the aorta
D. Narrowing of the aorta, which restricts left ventricular outflow

5 In a child with TOF, cyanosis results from:

A. A left-to-right shunt through a ventricular septal defect
B. A right-to-left shunt through a ventricular septal defect
C. An increase in pulmonary blood flow
D. A left-to-right shunt through a Blalock-Taussig shunt

6 When discussing TOF with the parents of a neonate diagnosed with this disorder, the nurse should:

A. Avoid medical jargon and highly technical explanations
B. Avoid repeating information
C. Avoid discussing any deformity, focusing instead on the child's attractive features
D. All of the above

SITUATION

Karen, age 9 months, has congenital heart disease. She is admitted to the hospital with a diagnosis of congestive heart failure (CHF) and is receiving digoxin.

Questions 7 to 11 refer to this situation.

7 Karen probably will exhibit which signs and symptoms associated with CHF?

A. Edema, bradycardia, increased urine output, and cyanosis
B. Dyspnea, edema, cyanosis, and bradycardia
C. Chest retractions, tachycardia, hypertension, and strong peripheral pulses
D. Tachycardia, dyspnea, gallop rhythm, and hepatomegaly

8 The nurse knows that digoxin, like other cardiac glycosides, can be extremely toxic. Which of the following is an early sign of digitalis toxicity?

A. Bradycardia
B. Increased activity
C. Respiratory distress
D. Tachycardia

9 When administering digoxin to Karen, the nurse should take all of the following actions *except:*

A. Monitoring the serum potassium level
B. Verifying the dosage with another nurse
C. Obtaining the apical heart rate before administration
D. Administering the medication with food

10 Karen is scheduled to undergo cardiac catheterization. Which nursing action takes the highest priority immediately after this procedure?

A. Obtaining a complete blood count
B. Increasing her oral fluid intake
C. Performing a neurologic assessment
D. Checking her vital signs

11 When assessing Karen after cardiac catheterization, the nurse notes that her affected extremity is cool to the touch and her nailbeds remain blanched during capillary refill evaluation. If these findings do not improve after 2 hours, the nurse should suspect:

A. Hematoma
B. Infection
C. Thrombosis
D. Hypothermia

SITUATION

Jennifer Gregory, age 3, is admitted to the hospital for corrective surgery for TOF. Until 3 months ago, she tolerated activity with minimal cyanosis and distress. At age 6 months, she underwent surgery to improve blood flow to the lungs.

Questions 12 to 14 refer to this situation.

12 During physical assessment, the nurse should expect all of the following findings in Jennifer *except:*

A. Toe clubbing
B. Heart murmur
C. Height and weight below the 50th percentile
D. Tachycardia

13 Before surgery, Jennifer has a "tet" or "blue" spell while crying, instinctively drawing herself into a knee-to-chest position. This position causes occlusion of the femoral arteries, leading to:

A. Increased systemic vascular resistance and increased pulmonary blood flow
B. Decreased systemic vascular resistance and increased pulmonary blood flow
C. Increased pulmonary vascular resistance and decreased pulmonary blood flow
D. Decreased pulmonary vascular resistance and increased pulmonary blood flow

14 Before discharge, the nurse helps Mrs. Gregory to plan low-sodium, high-protein meals for Jennifer. Which food would best meet these criteria?

A. Macaroni with cheese
B. Canned tomato soup
C. Hot dog
D. Homemade hamburger

SITUATION

Paul, age 8 months, is admitted to the pediatric intensive care unit after open-heart surgery. He is connected to a cardiac-respiratory monitor and is receiving humidified oxygen by Oxyhood. A central venous pressure line, a chest tube, and an indwelling urinary (Foley) catheter are in place.

Questions 15 to 17 refer to this situation.

15 Which clinical finding or laboratory result indicates that Paul is in renal failure?

A. Decreased blood urea nitrogen level
B. Decreased serum creatinine level
C. Oliguria
D. Polyuria

16 Early on the second postoperative day, Paul has an axillary temperature of 100° F (37.8° C). This finding may be a response to:

A. Hypothermic procedures
B. Anesthesia
C. Inflammation
D. Infection

17 Which nursing action is appropriate when caring for Paul's chest tube?

A. Ensuring that emergency clamps are available at the bedside
B. Opening the chest tube system to allow for maximum drainage
C. Notifying the surgeon if fluctuation in the water-seal chamber decreases
D. Checking the color and quantity of drainage at every shift

---

SITUATION

Ned, born 8 hours ago, is transported to a cardiac specialty hospital with an admitting diagnosis of tricuspid atresia based on echocardiogram findings. Arterial and venous umbilical catheters are in place—one to infuse a maintenance solution, the other to administer prostaglandin E.

One hour after admission, Ned undergoes cardiac catheterization. The physician confirms the diagnosis of tricuspid atresia, then performs a Raskind balloon septostomy. After surgery, Ned is admitted to the pediatric intensive care unit.

Questions 18 and 19 refer to this situation.

18 Tricuspid atresia is associated with which finding?

A. Ventricular arrhythmia
B. Cyanosis
C. Atrial arrhythmia
D. Increased arterial oxygen tension

19 Ned is receiving prostaglandin E, a vasodilator, to:

A. Maintain a patent ductus arteriosus
B. Keep the foramen ovale open
C. Increase right-to-left shunting of blood
D. Maintain systemic perfusion

SITUATION

Victor, age 10, visits the pediatrician for a routine preschool checkup. On physical examination, the pediatrician notes bilaterally weak femoral and popliteal pulses and no palpable posterior tibial or dorsalis pedis pulses. Blood pressure measures 40 mm Hg higher in the upper extremities than the lower extremities. The pediatrician suspects coarctation of the aorta and admits Victor to the hospital for testing. After test results confirm the diagnosis, Victor is scheduled for surgery to repair the defect.

Questions 20 and 21 refer to this situation.

20 Nursing assessment of Victor should include:

A. Observing the cardiac monitor for ventricular arrhythmias
B. Measuring blood pressure in all four extremities
C. Monitoring for seizures
D. Measuring blood pressure in the upper extremities only

21 Postoperatively, Victor will require all of the following nursing interventions *except:*

A. Hourly monitoring of blood pressure
B. Assessment of all pulses every 1 to 2 hours
C. Assessment of abdominal status every 2 to 4 hours
D. Maintenance of reverse isolation

SITUATION

Cindy, delivered 3 days ago at 28 weeks' gestation, develops a heart murmur. The physician diagnoses patent ductus arteriosus (PDA) and orders I.V. fluid administration and intubation on a mechanical ventilator.

Questions 22 to 24 refer to this situation.

22 In a healthy full-term neonate, the ductus arteriosus closes how soon after delivery?

A. 1 day
B. 3 days
C. 4 days
D. 7 days

23 Nursing assessment of Cindy should include:

A. Palpating peripheral pulses
B. Assessing the heart rate
C. Auscultating the chest
D. All of the above

24 Which nursing intervention is *not* appropriate for Cindy?

A. Monitoring fluid intake and output
B. Increasing external stimuli
C. Auscultating breath sounds
D. Monitoring arterial blood gas values

Answer sheet

	A	B	C	D
1	○	○	○	○
2	○	○	○	○
3	○	○	○	○
4	○	○	○	○
5	○	○	○	○
6	○	○	○	○
7	○	○	○	○
8	○	○	○	○
9	○	○	○	○
10	○	○	○	○
11	○	○	○	○
12	○	○	○	○
13	○	○	○	○
14	○	○	○	○
15	○	○	○	○
16	○	○	○	○
17	○	○	○	○
18	○	○	○	○
19	○	○	○	○
20	○	○	○	○
21	○	○	○	○
22	○	○	○	○
23	○	○	○	○
24	○	○	○	○

Answers and rationales

1 Correct answer—**D**

Endocarditis is an infection of the lining and valves of the heart caused by bacterial microorganisms. Bacteria entering the bloodstream—usually from a localized infection—grow on the heart's lining in areas of turbulent or disturbed blood flow. Maintaining good dental care helps prevent endocarditis by reducing the risk of bacteria entering the bloodstream. Invasive procedures do not increase the risk of endocarditis in a child with congenital heart disease who is receiving prophylactic antibiotics. Routine immunizations also do not increase the risk. Continuous antibiotic therapy is not recommended because microorganisms can become resistant to antibiotics.

2 Correct answer—**D**

Polycythemia—an increase in the number of red blood cells (RBCs)—is stimulated by chronic hypoxia associated with congenital heart disease. Overabundance of RBCs makes the blood more viscous, increasing the risk of cerebrovascular accident (CVA). RBCs may block vessels in the brain, causing vessel rupture or ischemia. Children with congenital heart disease have altered pulmonary blood flow caused by anatomic deviations; most have decreased exercise tolerance from insufficient nutritional intake and increased metabolic demands. However, altered pulmonary blood flow and decreased exercise tolerance do not cause CVA. Cardiomegaly—hypertrophy of the heart muscle—may result from heart failure or congenital heart disease; it is not associated with CVA.

3 Correct answer—**B**

A child with coarctation of the aorta—congenital narrowing of the aorta—has bounding pulses and high blood pressure in areas of the body receiving blood from vessels proximal to the defect. A child with patent ductus arteriosus typically has a wide pulse pressure caused by a low diastolic pressure from the shunting of blood. A child with aortic stenosis typically shows no symptoms except for a possible systolic heart murmur. A child with atrial septal defect typically has a harsh systolic murmur.

4 Correct answer—C

Tetralogy of Fallot (TOF) is characterized by four defects—pulmonary stenosis, right ventricular hypertrophy, ventricular septal defect, and dextroposition of the aorta. TOF is the most common cyanotic heart defect in children. Origination of the aorta from the right ventricle and origination of the pulmonary artery from the left ventricle characterizes transposition of the great vessels. A hole in the ventricular septum characterizes ventricular septal defect. Narrowing of the aorta occurs in aortic stenosis.

5 Correct answer—B

A right-to-left shunt through a ventricular septal defect forces desaturated blood to enter the systemic circulation, decreasing arterial oxygen tension and causing cyanosis (bluish skin discoloration). In TOF, decreased pulmonary blood flow combined with a right-to-left shunt causes cyanosis. The Blalock-Taussig procedure is a temporary surgical procedure used to treat hypoxic episodes; it is not the cause of cyanosis, but rather a temporary measure to correct it.

6 Correct answer—A

Health team members must convey consistent information in terms that the child's parents can understand. Medical jargon and technical explanations may be confusing and overwhelming to them. Because they may be experiencing anxiety, shock, or guilt, the nurse may need to repeat points that are unclear or may have been misunderstood. TOF is characterized by structural defects or deformities; these deformities must be discussed if the parents are to understand the child's disorder and its management.

7 Correct answer—D

Congestive heart failure (CHF) is a condition in which the heart cannot pump sufficient amounts of blood through the circulatory system to meet metabolic needs. Diminished cardiac output manifests as weak peripheral pulses and decreased blood pressure; decreased blood flow to the kidneys leads to decreased urine output. The body attempts to compensate for reduced cardiac output by activating the sympathetic nervous system, causing tachycardia, and by inducing the renal system to retain sodium and water. Because the heart cannot handle the increased blood volume, systemic congestion results. Hepatomegaly and edema are signs of systemic congestion. Increased blood volume also causes the ventricles to dilate, producing extra heart sounds described as gallop rhythm. As the left ventricle decompensates, capillary pressure increases; this leads to decreased lung compliance, evidenced by dyspnea and chest retractions. Cyanosis results from impaired respiratory gas exchange.

8 Correct answer—A

Bradycardia and vomiting are early signs of digitalis toxicity. In excessive blood drug levels, digoxin depresses sinoatrial node automaticity, markedly slowing the heart rate. Vomiting results from stimulation of the emetic control center in the medulla. Other symptoms of digitalis toxicity include visual disturbances (yellow-green halos), headache, and fatigue. Increased activity and respiratory distress are not indicative of digitalis toxicity.

9 Correct answer—D

Digoxin should not be administered with food because failure to consume all of the food may result in inaccurate drug intake. Digoxin should be administered at regular intervals 1 to 2 hours after meals. The nurse should monitor serum potassium levels because hypokalemia can increase digitalis toxicity. Because of the narrow margin between digoxin's therapeutic and toxic effects, the nurse always should verify the dosage with another nurse. To assess for arrhythmias, especially bradycardia, the nurse must obtain an apical heart rate before administering digoxin.

10 Correct answer—D

The nurse should check vital signs every 15 minutes after cardiac catheterization by checking the heart rate for 1 minute to detect bradycardia or arrhythmias, checking the pulses for equality, and checking blood pressure for hypotension (which may indicate hemorrhage). A complete blood count is obtained before cardiac catheterization and may not be necessary afterward. Because Karen has had no oral intake, the nurse should encourage oral fluid intake; however, this is not a priority because she still may be receiving an I.V. infusion as a source of hydration. Neurologic assessment is not required after cardiac catheterization.

11 Correct answer—C

Thrombi can form in the vasculature from injury to vessel walls during catheterization. A thrombus may occlude or partially block an artery, decreasing perfusion to the affected extremity. Altered arterial perfusion manifests as cool skin temperature, mottled skin, blanching, and diminished or absent peripheral pulses. Warm, pink extremities with strong pulses indicate good arterial perfusion. Hematoma is assessed by observing the puncture site for redness, swelling, and induration. Infection is not apparent immediately after catheterization and would not affect the pulse rate. Hypothermia is assessed by taking the child's temperature.

12 Correct answer—A

TOF is a cyanotic congenital heart disease. Clubbing of fingers, not toes, is a sign of chronic oxygen deprivation; it would be expected in a child who has had compromised tissue oxygenation since birth. Heart murmur also is likely because a heart defect causes turbulent blood flow. Children with congenital heart disease typically experience below-average growth from feeding problems and increased oxygen demands. The heart attempts to meet the body's oxygen needs by increasing the rate of contractions, resulting in tachycardia.

13 Correct answer—A

Cyanotic heart disease reduces pulmonary blood flow. Many children with such disease adopt a knee-to-chest position because it is a natural shunting maneuver that channels more blood to the lungs. This position increases systemic vascular resistance by minimizing the routing of poorly oxygenated blood to the general circulation and maximizing pulmonary blood flow.

14 Correct answer—D

A child with congenital heart disease may require dietary sodium restriction if the disease causes fluid retention, which increases the heart's workload. Because protein is essential to growth, a high-protein intake is encouraged for a child such as Jennifer who commonly demonstrates below-average growth. Homemade hamburgers and other nonprocessed meats are low in sodium and high in protein. Cheese is a poor choice because it is high in sodium.

Canned soups also have a high sodium content. Hot dogs and other processed meats contain moderate to high sodium levels.

15 Correct answer—C

Renal failure may result from preexisting renal disease and a period of low cardiac output. In renal failure, clinical findings and laboratory results include oliguria (urine output below 1 ml/kg/hour) and elevated blood urea nitrogen (BUN) and serum creatinine levels. BUN and creatinine are metabolic waste products normally excreted via the urine; elevated levels indicate accumulation of these by-products from renal dysfunction.

16 Correct answer—C

For 24 to 48 hours after surgery, body temperature may rise to 100° F (37.7° C) or slightly higher from inflammation, which is a normal response to surgical tissue manipulation and trauma. After 48 hours, an above-normal temperature usually signals infection. Hypothermia and anesthesia cause a temperature decrease.

17 Correct answer—A

A chest tube is inserted to remove secretions and air from the pleural space so that the lungs can reexpand. When caring for a patient with a chest tube, the nurse should ensure that emergency clamps are available at the bedside because the chest tube must be clamped if the integrity of the tube or drainage system is compromised. The system is airtight and should never be opened because air entering the tube may travel into the pleural space, causing pneumothorax. Decreased fluctuation in the water-seal chamber is expected because it indicates lung expansion. The nurse should monitor the color and quantity of drainage hourly, not at every shift. Initially, drainage is bright red but later becomes serous. Increased drainage (more than 3 ml/kg/hour for 3 hours) may indicate hemorrhage.

18 Correct answer—B

In tricuspid atresia, blood cannot pass from the right atrium to the right ventricle and therefore cannot reach the lungs, making gas exchange impossible. As right atrial pressure increases, blood is shunted from the right atrium through the foreman ovale to the left atrium. Such right-to-left shunting causes mixing of oxygen-poor blood with systemic blood in the left atrium, lowering arterial oxygen tension. The mixture of saturated and desaturated blood enters the circulatory system—already experiencing decreased pulmonary blood flow. The result is cyanosis. Neither ventricular nor atrial arrhythmias may appear on initial assessment, whereas cyanosis always is present.

19 Correct answer—A

Because prostaglandin E causes vasodilation and relaxes smooth muscle, it is administered to maintain a patent ductus arteriosus (PDA), a wide muscular vessel connecting the pulmonary artery with the aorta. In fetal circulation, the ductus arteriosus allows right-to-left shunting from the pulmonary artery to the aorta, decreasing blood flow to the nonfunctioning lungs. After birth, this passage becomes nonfunctional and eventually disappears. In tricuspid atresia, the ductus arteriosus remains open, permitting left-to-right shunting. Prostaglandin E acts on the smooth muscle of this structure, maintaining its patency until a more reliable surgical anastomosis can be established. No evidence indicates that Ned has a patent foramen ovale.

20 Correct answer—B

In coarctation of the aorta, or narrowing of the aorta, blood pressure is higher in the upper extremities than the lower extremities. Cardiac monitoring is not indicated because coarctation of the aorta rarely is associated with arrhythmias. Seizures rarely occur as complications of this disorder. Measuring blood pressure only in the upper extremities does not provide comprehensive data to assess systemic circulation and perfusion.

21 Correct answer—D

Because Victor is not receiving medication that would increase his risk of infection, reverse (protective) isolation is not indicated. The nurse should monitor Victor's blood pressure hourly to evaluate his cardiopulmonary status and check his pulses every 1 to 2 hours to evaluate his arterial perfusion status. Abdominal assessment also is necessary because mesenteric ischemia is a potential postoperative complication; in this assessment, the nurse auscultates bowel sounds, palpates for abdominal tenderness, and notes any abdominal distention.

22 Correct answer—A

Immediately after birth, fetal circulation begins the transition to newborn circulation. The ductus arteriosus constricts in response to increased oxygen in the pulmonary artery and the presence of prostaglandins. This process usually is completed within 24 hours; however, complete closure of the ductus arteriosus takes several months. Premature neonates have an increased incidence of PDA and many suffer severe respiratory disease associated with decreased arterial oxygen tension. The latter may allow the ductus arteriosus to remain open or reopen.

23 Correct answer—D

In neonates with persistent PDA, blood is shunted from the aorta to the pulmonary artery, then recirculates through the left atrium and left ventricle. This increases the cardiac work load and exacerbates pulmonary vascular congestion. CHF develops because the heart cannot compensate for the increased work load. In a neonate with PDA, peripheral pulses may increase in amplitude (above 25 mm Hg). When auscultating for heart rate and heart sounds, the nurse should hear a characteristic machinery-type murmur—a result of blood flowing from the aorta through the PDA. (However, this murmur may be absent in a premature neonate because normally high pulmonary resistance in the pulmonary artery tends to equalize the pressure between this artery and the aorta, minimizing the amount of blood shunted.

24 Correct answer—B

The nurse must limit external stimuli because stress can increase oxygen consumption and reduce cardiac and pulmonary efficiency in a neonate with PDA. Because PDA commonly causes CHF, the nurse should monitor Cindy's fluid intake and output; decreased cardiac output may cause fluid retention. The nurse also should auscultate breath sounds for deviations that may signal infection or fluid accumulation. Arterial blood gas values help assess impaired gas exchange.

CHAPTER 14

Neurologic and Musculoskeletal Disorders

Questions

1 Decorticate posturing is characterized by:

A. Adduction of the arms at the shoulders
B. Abduction of the arms at the shoulders
C. Extension of the wrists
D. Flexion of the legs at the knees

2 Which term refers to involuntary muscle contraction and relaxation?

A. Reflex
B. Seizure
C. Subluxation
D. Hypotonia

3 For lumbar puncture, an infant should be placed in:

A. An arched, side-lying position with the neck flexed onto the chest
B. An arched, side-lying position that avoids flexion of the neck onto the chest
C. A mummy restraint
D. A prone position with the head over the edge of the table or bed

4 Neonates with subarachnoid hemorrhage most commonly have:

A. Overwhelming central nervous system deterioration
B. Pallor and an abnormally low hematocrit
C. Seizures but an otherwise healthy status
D. Hypotonia and fixed pupils

5 Encephalitis may arise as a complication after any of the following systemic viral illnesses *except:*

A. Cytomegalovirus
B. Mumps
C. Measles
D. Varicella

6 Nursing care for a child with increased intracranial pressure includes:

A. Elevating the head of the bed 60 degrees
B. Avoiding neck vein compression
C. Performing vigorous range-of-motion exercises
D. Performing chest percussion

7 Common signs of meningitis include fever, poor feeding, vomiting, and:

A. Pallor
B. Vesicular lesions
C. Sunken fontanels
D. Seizures

8 Which of the following is a potential complication of meningitis?

A. Central circulatory collapse
B. Inappropriate secretion of antidiuretic hormone
C. Speech impairment
D. Growth retardation

9 Nursing care for a child with bacterial meningitis should include:

A. Instituting respiratory isolation
B. Implementing universal precautions
C. Administering oral antibiotics, as prescribed
D. Administering furosemide (Lasix), as prescribed

10 Reye's syndrome is associated with:

A. Parasitic infection
B. Bacterial infection
C. Viral infection
D. Chlamydial infection

11 Cerebrospinal fluid is produced mainly by the:

A. Arachnoid layer of the meninges
B. Arteries in the circle of Willis
C. Choroid plexus of the ventricles
D. Vital centers of the medulla oblongata

12 Meningomyelocele must be repaired as soon as possible to prevent which problem?

A. Motor paralysis from trauma to the spinal cord or nerve root caused by pressure on the back
B. Spontaneous rupture or ulceration of the protruding sac, with subsequent meningitis
C. Extrusion of additional spinal cord or nerve tissue into the sac during movement
D. Massive hemorrhage from exposed spinal blood vessels

13 Preoperative nursing care for an infant who is scheduled for surgical repair of meningomyelocele includes:

A. Providing parental support
B. Keeping the protruding sac dry
C. Picking the infant up for feeding while protecting the protruding sac
D. All of the above

SITUATION

Denise Allen, born 10 days ago, has congenital dislocation of both hips and bilateral clubfoot. She is placed in a bilateral hip spica cast.

Questions 14 to 16 refer to this situation.

14 When assessing Denise for congenital hip dislocation, the nurse may note all of the following signs *except:*

A. Asymmetry of the gluteal folds
B. Limited abduction on the affected side
C. A characteristic limp when placed in a standing position
D. An audible click when abducting the hips

15 To treat congenital hip dislocation, the head of the femur is placed in the acetabulum and maintained there. The legs should be maintained in which position?

A. Adducted and extended
B. Abducted and extended
C. Adducted and flexed
D. Abducted and flexed

16 When preparing Denise's parents for her discharge, the nurse should advise them that:

A. They should avoid holding Denise to prevent trauma to the cast
B. Denise should not be breast-fed because of cast restrictions
C. The hip spica cast cannot be kept dry if Denise does not achieve bladder and bowel control
D. They should notify the physician if Denise's toes become edematous or discolored or if she cannot move them

---

SITUATION

Pauline, age 14, was diagnosed with scoliosis 3 years ago. Because the disorder has progressed significantly during the past 2 years, the physician admits her to the pediatric hospital for spinal fusion and casting.

Questions 17 and 18 refer to this situation.

17 Which observation is most typical in a patient with scoliosis?

A. The patient limps when walking
B. The patient has difficulty lying flat
C. The patient has an uneven hemline or unequal pant lengths
D. The patient has numbness or tingling in the feet

18 Which remark would be appropriate for the nurse to make when teaching Pauline about her upcoming surgery?

A. "I realize you must be nervous. You shouldn't worry because we'll take care of you completely"
B. "This surgery will not slow you down. You'll be active before you know it"
C. "You'll share a room with another adolescent so you can help each other"
D. "You must be worried about your appearance. This surgery will straighten your back so you can perform many of your daily activities"

SITUATION

Tony, a 16-year-old high school junior, has an accident while riding a motor bike. He is admitted to the hospital with a fractured right femur and multiple bruises and abrasions of the arm, face, and chest. Buck's extension traction is applied to his right leg, and he is scheduled for surgery in 48 hours.

Questions 19 to 22 refer to this situation.

19 For the first 24 hours after Tony's admission, the nurse should assess Tony's right thigh and buttock because:

A. He will complain of discomfort at the fracture site
B. A large amount of blood may be lost into the tissue
C. The fracture site is prone to infection
D. Trauma initially causes loss of muscle tone

20 While Tony is in Buck's extension traction, the nurse should inform him that the head of his bed should not be raised more than 30 degrees because this will:

A. Cause postural hypotension
B. Strain the pull of the traction
C. Induce vomiting
D. Reduce countertraction

21 Which nursing intervention is most likely to promote Tony's skin integrity?

A. Applying a footboard
B. Performing passive range-of-motion exercises
C. Administering a back rub during every shift
D. Providing high-calcium snacks

22 When preparing Tony to walk on crutches, the nurse should teach him exercises to develop his:

A. Ankle extensors
B. Arm flexors
C. Abdominal muscles
D. Hamstring muscles

SITUATION

Marisa, age 12, fell 5 days ago in gym class and now complains of swelling, warmth, and tenderness of the left leg. The physician diagnoses osteomyelitis of the left femur and admits her to the hospital.

Questions 23 to 25 refer to this situation.

23 The most important *initial* nursing action when caring for Marisa is to:

A. Administer I.V. antibiotic therapy, as ordered
B. Draw blood for cultures, as ordered
C. Monitor hepatic and renal studies
D. Prepare her for immediate surgery, as ordered

24 During the acute phase of osteomyelitis, which nursing intervention is most appropriate?

A. Encouraging ambulation on crutches
B. Referring the patient to a physical therapist to prevent contractures
C. Encouraging weight bearing on the affected limb
D. Controlling pain and handling the affected limb gently

25 Which action is the nurse's highest priority when Marisa starts antibiotic therapy?

A. Maintaining I.V. antibiotic therapy, as prescribed, until blood cultures are negative
B. Explaining to her parents why I.V. antibiotic therapy must continue for 2 to 3 weeks
C. Preparing her for immediate discharge and scheduling follow-up visits
D. Discontinuing the medication, as prescribed, as soon as bone pain dissipates

---

SITUATION

Roberta Schwinn, age 14 months, is referred to the child development center for evaluation of speech impairment, drooling, and spasticity of all her extremities. The physician makes a preliminary diagnosis of the spastic quadriplegia form of cerebral palsy.

Questions 26 to 29 refer to this situation.

26 Roberta's mother tells the nurse she is afraid Roberta will die as her nervous system deteriorates. The nurse should explain that:

A. Cerebral palsy is a slow, progressive neurologic disorder that rarely results in death
B. Cerebral palsy is a chronic, nonprogressive neurologic disorder of muscle coordination resulting from brain injury that rarely is fatal
C. Cerebral palsy represents a group of neuromuscular dysfunctions, and further testing is required to establish a prognosis
D. Cerebral palsy is the most common permanent physical disability of childhood, and the prognosis depends on the underlying cause

27 Conditions that have been proposed as causes of cerebral palsy include:

A. Premature birth and perinatal asphyxia
B. Intracranial hemorrhage and spherocytosis
C. Bronchopulmonary dysplasia and Guillain-Barré syndrome
D. Ischemia and pulmonary stenosis

28 In a child with the spastic quadriplegia form of cerebral palsy, increased tension on the hip adductors, hip internal rotators, and calf muscles causes which abnormality?

A. Hip dislocation
B. Knock-knee deformity
C. Marked leg bowing
D. Scissoring and toe pointing

29 Which nursing action would offer the most support for Robert's parents?

A. Encouraging Roberta's early and continuous participation in a special school program
B. Helping the family to plan for Roberta's future needs
C. Assessing for developmental changes during subsequent visits
D. Helping the family to meet Roberta's current needs

SITUATION

Joel, age 11, is admitted to the pediatric rehabilitation unit after orthopedic surgery to the lower extremities to release contractures and maintain independent ambulation. He was diagnosed with Duchenne's muscular dystrophy at age 4 after showing signs of muscle weakness, followed by an abnormal gait and Gowers' sign (rising from the floor in a sitting or squatting position).

Questions 30 to 32 refer to this situation.

30 Diagnosis of Duchenne's muscular dystrophy is confirmed by:

A. Muscle biopsy showing hypertrophy of muscle fibers
B. Electromyography revealing an increase in amplitude
C. Serum enzyme studies
D. Pulmonary function tests

31 Which nursing intervention would help prevent muscle atrophy during Joel's postoperative recovery?

A. Using bracing with a rigid corset for support
B. Referring him for physical therapy
C. Performing postural drainage and pulmonary toilet
D. Scheduling ambulation periods of at least 3 hours a day

32 Which nursing intervention is most appropriate for a patient with muscular dystrophy who has a nursing diagnosis of *Impaired physical mobility related to muscle wasting and weakness?*

A. Encouraging deep breathing and coughing
B. Providing small, frequent, and easily digested meals
C. Providing learning opportunities for home exercises
D. Allowing time for self-help activities

SITUATION

Glenn, age 3 months, was born with hydrocephalus. He underwent surgery for placement of a ventriculoperitoneal shunt at age 2 months. He was just admitted to the pediatric unit for shunt revision (operative replacement or repair of the shunt) after the shunt tubing became obstructed by particulate matter.

Questions 33 to 35 refer to this situation.

33 Hydrocephalus may result from:

A. Excessive growth of cranial bones and brain tissue
B. Secretion of an abnormal substance in the brain
C. Obstruction of the ventricles, preventing resorption of cerebro-spinal fluid
D. Lack of prenatal brain development caused by a genetically acquired defect

34 Glenn has increased intracranial pressure (ICP) from the shunt obstruction. Signs of increased ICP include all of the following *except:*

A. Increasing head size
B. Poor feeding
C. High-pitched crying
D. Depressed fontanels

35 The immediate postoperative plan of care for Glenn should include which nursing action?

A. Maintaining fluid and electrolyte balance through I.V. fluid regulation
B. Maintaining him in a prone position at all times
C. Keeping him sedated to promote rest and healing
D. Avoiding handling to prevent trauma to the incision site

SITUATION

Alison, age 12, is admitted to the hospital for a workup after recent onset of generalized tonic-clonic seizures. The physician prescribes anticonvulsants, which curb the seizures. Five days after her admission, Alison is scheduled for discharge.

Questions 36 and 37 refer to this situation.

36 Which statement about generalized tonic-clonic seizures is correct?

A. They are triggered by electrical hyperactivity throughout the brain, not just in a localized or confined area
B. They usually are preceded by tingling sensations and flashes of light
C. They are over in about 30 seconds, do not cause loss of consciousness, and have a specific electrical activity center
D. They are characterized by a brief loss of consciousness with little or no change in muscle tone

37 The physician prescribes phenytoin (Dilantin) for Alison to take after discharge. Which side effect may occur with use of this drug?

A. Vitamin K deficiency
B. Gum hyperplasia
C. Diarrhea
D. Hypertension

Answer sheet

	A B C D		A B C D
1	○○○○	31	○○○○
2	○○○○	32	○○○○
3	○○○○	33	○○○○
4	○○○○	34	○○○○
5	○○○○	35	○○○○
6	○○○○	36	○○○○
7	○○○○	37	○○○○
8	○○○○		
9	○○○○		
10	○○○○		
11	○○○○		
12	○○○○		
13	○○○○		
14	○○○○		
15	○○○○		
16	○○○○		
17	○○○○		
18	○○○○		
19	○○○○		
20	○○○○		
21	○○○○		
22	○○○○		
23	○○○○		
24	○○○○		
25	○○○○		
26	○○○○		
27	○○○○		
28	○○○○		
29	○○○○		
30	○○○○		

Answers and rationales

1 Correct answer—**A**

Decorticate posturing, a sign of cerebral cortex dysfunction, is characterized by adduction of the arms at the shoulders. The arms and wrists are flexed and form fists on the chest; the legs are adducted and extended.

2 Correct answer—**B**

A seizure is defined as involuntary muscle contraction and relaxation. The terms *seizure* and *convulsion* often are used interchangeably. A seizure disorder may result from idiopathic (unknown) or acquired causes. Brain injury, infections, and biochemical disturbances may trigger acquired seizure disorders. A reflex is a response to a given stimulus. Subluxation refers to partial dislocation of a joint. Hypotonia is an abnormal decrease in muscle strength.

3 Correct answer—**B**

For lumbar puncture, an infant should be placed in an arched position to maximize the space between the L3 and L5 vertebrae. The nurse's hands should rest on the back of the infant's shoulders to prevent neck flexion, which could block the airway and cause respiratory arrest. The infant should be at the edge of the bed or table during the procedure, and the nurse should speak quietly to calm him. A mummy restraint limits access to the lumbar area because it involves snugly wrapping the child's trunk and extremities in a blanket or towel; this restraint is appropriate for procedures involving the head or neck because it leaves only these body parts exposed. A prone position would not separate the vertebral spaces.

4 Correct answer—**C**

Most neonates with subarachnoid hemorrhage exhibit seizures but otherwise are healthy. Seizures usually begin on the second day after birth. Hemorrhage—venous in origin and usually self-limited—arises secondary to hypoxia or trauma.

5 Correct answer—**A**

Encephalitis (inflammation of the brain) may result from direct invasion of the central nervous system (CNS) by a virus or postinfectious CNS involvement after a viral infection. Causative viruses include mumps, measles, varicella, arbovirus, herpesviruses, and enteroviruses. Cytomegalovirus is transmitted prenatally and is not associated with encephalitis.

6 Correct answer—**B**

The nurse should avoid neck vein compression because this interferes with venous return and may exacerbate increased intracranial pressure (ICP). The bed should be elevated 15 to 30 degrees, with the child's head in a midline position to promote venous return. Mild range-of-motion exercises are indicated, and external stimuli should be minimized to help reduce ICP. Chest percussion and suctioning should be avoided because they increase ICP.

7 Correct answer—**D**

Seizures and irritability are common signs of meningitis. A bulging fontanel may appear in infants and young children. An older child may complain of headache and photophobia. A petechial rash may develop. Nuchal rigidity sometimes occurs depending on the child's age (it rarely occurs in children under age 2). Vesicular lesions are not associated with meningitis. Pallor may be indicative of any problem and is not specific to meningitis.

8 Correct answer—**B**

Meningitis may cause long-term complications or death from peripheral circulatory collapse. CNS injury or inflammation commonly results in hypothalamic dysfunction, which leads to inappropriate secretion of antidiuretic hormone—a condition causing fluid retention and serum hypotonicity. In turn, serum hypotonicity and hypervolemia result in cerebral edema. Impaired vision and hearing, cerebral palsy, mental retardation, seizures, and cognitive disabilities are other potential complications of meningitis. Speech impairment and growth retardation are not associated with this illness.

9 Correct answer—**A**

Respiratory isolation is indicated because bacterial meningitis is transmitted via nasopharyngeal droplets. The child must be placed in a private room; all persons entering the room must wear a mask. Gown and gloves must be worn when providing direct care. Universal precautions are not adequate to prevent transmission of bacterial meningitis because they do not mandate wearing a mask. Antibiotics are administered I.V., with special measures used to maintain the I.V. line for an extended period. For example, the child may nccd to be restrained to prevent dislodgment of the I.V. device. During play, protective coverings or conversion to a heparin lock may help preserve the integrity of the I.V. device. Children with meningitis commonly have an intravascular fluid volume deficit from fever, vomiting, and diarrhea; consequently, furosemide (Lasix) is not administered because it may exacerbate this deficit.

10 Correct answer—C

Reye's syndrome, or toxic encephalopathy, commonly follows viral influenza or varicella infection in children. Although its etiology is unclear, the disorder is linked to aspirin ingestion. Children ages 6 to 11 most commonly are affected.

11 Correct answer—C

Presumably, the main site of cerebrospinal fluid (CSF) formation is the choroid plexus of the lateral ventricles. Some CSF also is produced by the brain parenchyma.

12 Correct answer—B

Meningomyelocele refers to protrusion of part of the meninges and spinal cord substance through a defect in the spinal column. Early repair of this defect offers the most favorable outcome because spontaneous rupture or ulceration of the protruding sac can lead to meningitis or death. Motor paralysis from trauma to the spinal cord or nerve root, extrusion of additional spinal cord or nerve tissue, and massive hemorrhage are unlikely because meticulous care usually is taken to avoid injury or pressure on the meningomyelocele area. For instance, the neonate is positioned on the side only—never on the back—before surgical repair.

13 Correct answer—A

For the parents, the birth of a neonate with a congenital defect represents loss of the healthy child they had anticipated. The nurse should encourage the parents to discuss their feelings and to grieve. Before surgery, the protruding sac must be kept moist using sterile nonadherent dressings. Picking the infant up for feeding is contraindicated; typically, the neonate is fed in a side-lying or prone position with the head to the side until the incision site heals.

14 Correct answer—C

The characteristic limp in children with congenital hip dislocation results from hip instability; it would not appear until the child begins to walk. Asymmetry of the gluteal folds, limited abduction on the affected side, shortening of the limb on the affected side, and an audible click when abducting the hips are signs of congenital hip dislocation that the nurse may note during physical assessment.

15 Correct answer—D

The head of the femur can be maintained in the desired position by abducting the hip, with the legs abducted and flexed. This position encourages deepening of the acetabulum so that it will become a more stable receptacle for the head of the femur. Stabilization is maintained by a Pavlik harness or hip spica cast.

16 Correct answer—D

Circulatory status must be monitored carefully after a cast is applied. Edema, discoloration, or inability to move distal extremities suggests circulatory impairment. Altered circulation to the affected extremity may impair bone healing and cause localized tissue damage. Parents should be taught to observe the neonate's limbs several times a day and to notify the physician if signs of impaired circulation arise. A neonate in a cast should be held in the same manner as other neonates to promote normal development. She can be breast-fed if pillows are used to support the immobilized extremity. Although the perineum of a neonate in a hip spica cast must be kept clean and dry to prevent skin breakdown and infection, bowel and bladder control is not required. The parents should be able to keep the perineal area clean and dry with frequent diaper changes.

17 Correct answer—C

Scoliosis is lateral curve of the spine; in about 80% of patients with this disorder, the cause is unknown. An uneven hemline, unequal pant lengths, rounded shoulders, prominence of one hip, and unequal shoulder-to-fingertip length may be observed. Adolescent idiopathic scoliosis, which affects more girls than boys, occurs in children ages 10 through 18—the age at which skeletal maturity is reached. The other options are atypical of a patient with scoliosis.

18 Correct answer—D

Adolescents are most concerned with body image, peer acceptance, and independence. The nurse should be truthful about how the surgery will affect the patient's appearance. After surgery, Pauline's spine will be straightened and will not bend further. She will appear taller and have better posture; after the cast is removed, she probably will have a nicely shaped body. Adolescents should be encouraged to care for themselves as much as possible.

19 Correct answer—B

Soft-tissue contusions commonly accompany fractures, especially fractures of the femur. Severe hemorrhage of these tissues may occur after injury. The nurse should expect the patient to complain of pain at the fracture site; the pain, which can be managed with analgesics, is not a sign of complications. Although infection is usually associated only with compound fractures (those in which the bone protrudes through the skin), the nurse should assess for infection postoperatively (not preoperatively) because surgical manipulation may introduce pathogens into the fracture site. After a fracture, the patient typically has muscle spasms (from increased muscle tone), which are relieved by traction and muscle relaxants.

20 Correct answer—D

Raising the head of the bed to a sitting position (more than 30 degrees) reduces the pull of the patient's weight; this decreases countertraction to the pull of weights applied to distal bone fragments. Reduced countertraction reduces the efficiency of traction in realigning bones and minimizing muscle spasms.

21 Correct answer—C

A patient in traction must remain supine for extended periods. Giving frequent backrubs stimulates blood supply to the back, shoulders, and buttocks—areas predisposed to skin breakdown in a bedridden patient. A footboard is used to help prevent foot drop. Range-of-motion exercises are performed to preserve joint function. High-calcium snacks may promote bone healing.

22 Correct answer—B

The arm flexors (shoulder girdle and upper extremity muscles) need strengthening so the patient can bear weight when walking with crutches. Exercises to strengthen and coordinate these muscle groups should begin as soon as the patient is ambulatory. Hamstring muscles, which flex the thigh, and ankle muscles, which extend the foot, do not need additional strengthening because they normally bear weight. Abdominal muscles play a minimal role in weight bearing.

23 Correct answer—B

Osteomyelitis, an infectious bone disease, begins in the metaphysis (growing portion) of the bone. Typically, it results from *Staphylococcus aureus* or *H. influenzae* infection. Before antibiotic therapy begins, blood cultures must be obtained to identify the pathogen and determine its sensitivity to antimicrobial agents. Treatment may include high doses of penicillin in combination with methicillin or oxacillin. Hepatic and renal studies are obtained during the course of antibiotic therapy to monitor for side effects of drugs. Surgery may be necessary later to drain abscesses.

24 Correct answer—D

Because osteomyelitis may be extremely painful, pain management and gentle handling of the affected limb are indicated. The patient is placed on complete bed rest and the affected extremity is immobilized to control infection. Ambulation, physical therapy, and weight bearing are not initiated until the infection subsides.

25 Correct answer—B

Long-term antibiotic therapy is required to prevent osteomyelitis recurrence and chronic bone deformities. The child is hospitalized for the duration of therapy—usually 2 to 3 weeks. Blood culture results may be negative even with bone infection. Medication is continued even if the patient does not have bone pain. The patient will be discharged with a prescription for oral antibiotics and instructions for close follow-up monitoring.

26 Correct answer—B

Cerebral palsy is a chronic, nonprogressive disorder of movement and posture resulting from a defect or lesion in the immature brain. Its etiology, clinical features, and course are variable but usually not life-threatening. Although cerebral palsy is the most common permanent physical disability of childhood, the prognosis for a normal life span is good and does not depend on the cause of the disorder or further testing.

27 Correct answer—A

Asphyxia and ischemia are the most common causes of cerebral palsy; premature, low-birth-weight neonates are particularly susceptible to intracranial bleeding and hypoxia, which can result in cerebral injury leading to cerebral palsy. Forces arising during labor can cause brain trauma in a premature neonate (as a result of the neonate's fragile state, increased capillary permeability, and prolonged prothrombin time). Spherocytosis, bronchopulmonary dysplasia, pulmonary stenosis, and Guillain-Barré syndrome do not cause cerebral palsy.

28 Correct answer—D

In a child with the spastic quadriplegia form of cerebral palsy, the thighs are extended at the hips, causing extension, internal rotation, and adduction of the legs. The feet usually are plantar-flexed at the ankles, resulting in scissoring and toe pointing.

29 Correct answer—D

Before parents can plan for the future, they must be able to care for the child today. Therefore, the nurse should address current child care needs first. Not all children with cerebral palsy require a special education program, although many do because of physical and intellectual limitations. Children with cerebral palsy typically exhibit developmental delays; although assessing for developmental changes at subsequent visits may provide encouragement for the parents about their child's progress, providing immediate support is the nurse's priority.

30 Correct answer—C

Duchenne's muscular dystrophy, the most common and severe form of muscular dystrophy in children, is an X-linked inherited disorder characterized by progressive muscle weakness and wasting. Generalized weakness progresses slowly until death occurs from respiratory or cardiac failure. Duchenne's muscular dystrophy is confirmed by serum enzyme studies—specifically, high levels of serum creatine phosphokinase, aldolase, and aspartate aminotransferase. Muscle biopsy reveals degenerating muscle fibers; electromyography shows a decrease in the amplitude and duration of motor unit potentials. Pulmonary function tests play no role in diagnosing muscular dystrophy.

31 Correct answer—D

Muscle atrophy caused by inactivity is common in immobilized patients. Having the patient walk at least 3 hours a day to maintain muscle strength is an appropriate nursing intervention. A patient with muscular dystrophy may require bracing with a rigid corset to support the spinal column; however, this does not prevent muscle atrophy. Physical therapy may be indicated to manage contractures that cannot be corrected by surgery; however, this is not the case in this situation. Postural drainage and pulmonary toilet are used to help prevent respiratory infections.

32 Correct answer—C

To maintain the patient's mobility and diminish muscle wasting and weakness, the nurse should provide opportunities for learning exercises that can be performed easily at home, such as passive and active range-of-motion exercises. The other answers may be appropriate for other nursing diagnoses. For example, deep breathing and coughing are used to maintain airway clearance, which is critical in preventing respiratory tract infections (which increase in frequency and severity as respiratory muscles deteriorate). Good nutrition promotes health and prevents such complications as obesity, which is related to mobility restrictions and excessive calorie consumption. Because many children with muscular dystrophy are withdrawn and passive, encouraging self-help activities maximizes independence.

33 Correct answer—C

Hydrocephalus occurs when the ventricles of the brain are obstructed, preventing circulation and resorption of CSF. Increased CSF causes ventricular dilation, leading to increased ICP. Hydrocephalus may result from excess CSF secretion or insufficient CSF resorption in the subarachnoid space. The head enlargement seen in neonates with hydrocephalus is caused by fluid accumulation and separation of cranial bones along suture lines—not from excessive growth of cranial bones and brain tissue. No abnormal substances are secreted in the brain. Hydrocephalus is not a genetic disorder.

34 Correct answer—D

Depressed fontanels are not an indication of increased ICP; they signal dehydration in an infant. A ventriculoperitoneal shunt allows CSF to drain from the brain; when the shunt is obstructed, CSF accumulates, causing increased ICP. Signs of increased ICP include increasing head size, dilated scalp veins, poor feeding, lethargy, irritability, high-pitched crying, and bulging fontanels.

35 Correct answer—A

After shunt revision, the infant usually is maintained on parenteral fluids for 24 to 48 hours. In a child with a ventriculoperitoneal shunt, oral feedings are restricted postoperatively until bowel sounds return. The patient usually is positioned on the nonsurgical side to prevent pressure on the shunt. The head of the bed can be flat or slightly elevated, depending on physician's orders. A flat position prevents CSF from draining too quickly; a slightly elevated position promotes drainage by gravity. Sedatives are contraindicated because the nurse must monitor the child's level of consciousness. Handling the child cannot be avoided completely.

36 Correct answer—A

Generalized tonic-clonic seizures are caused by uncontrolled electrical hyperactivity in the brain; they have no specific focal point or location and occur without warning. They rarely are preceded by sensorimotor effects, such as tingling sensations or flashes of light. Loss of consciousness is immediate, followed by tonic (contraction) muscle activity. The tonic phase lasts approximately 20 to 30 seconds and is followed by a clonic (relaxation) phase lasting approximately 30 seconds. After the seizure, the patient typically is confused and drowsy. Focal seizures occur in distinct areas of the brain—most commonly the frontal, temporal, and parietal lobes. Absence seizures are characterized by a brief loss of consciousness, with little or no change in muscle tone.

37 Correct answer—B

Phenytoin (Dilantin) is associated with such side effects as gum hyperplasia, hirsutism, rash, ataxia, vitamin D and folate deficiencies, anorexia, nausea, vomiting, constipation, and hypotension.

CHAPTER 15

Hematologic Disorders

Questions

1 The normal hematocrit for a full-term neonate is:

A. 30% to 35%
B. 35% to 45%
C. 55% to 65%
D. 65% to 75%

2 The nurse should expect which laboratory or clinical findings in a 9-month-old infant with sickle cell anemia?

A. Painful symmetrical swelling of the hands and feet
B. Gangrenous leg ulcers
C. Normal hemoglobin level and hematocrit
D. Fine macular rash

3 All of the following conditions predispose a neonate to hyperbilirubinemia *except:*

A. Enclosed hemorrhage
B. ABO blood incompatibility
C. Sepsis
D. Bottle-feeding

4 Discharge preparation for the parents of a child who has undergone splenectomy should include all of the following *except:*

A. Instructing them to notify the physician if the child has a fever
B. Informing them that the child will be prescribed oral penicillin indefinitely
C. Ensuring them that the child is not at risk for overwhelming infection because pneumococcal vaccine was administered before surgery
D. Explaining the importance of having the child wear a medical identification tag

---

SITUATION

Ron, age 15 months, is brought to the pediatric clinic for a well-child checkup. Routine testing reveals a hemoglobin level of 6.8 g/dl and a hematocrit of 21.1%. Further testing confirms that Ron has iron-deficiency anemia.

Questions 5 to 7 refer to this situation.

5 Which disorder causes accumulation of hemoglobin precursors similar to that in iron-deficiency anemia?

A. Lead poisoning
B. Hemophilia
C. Aplastic anemia
D. Idiopathic thrombocytic purpura

6 Oral iron therapy may cause all of the following side effects *except:*

A. Gastric irritation
B. Pica
C. Blackened stools
D. Darkened teeth

7 To promote absorption of the iron supplement, the nurse should instruct Ron's mother to administer the supplement to him:

A. During meals
B. Two hours after meals, with orange juice
C. Two hours after meals, with milk
D. Immediately before meals

SITUATION

Vanessa Billings, a 10-year-old patient with sickle cell disease, is admitted to the hospital with a fever and joint pain. On admission, vital sign assessment reveals a temperature of 102° F (38.8° C), a pulse rate of 110 beats/minute, a respiratory rate of 36 breaths/ minute, and blood pressure of 130/86 mm Hg. Twenty-four hours later, Vanessa lies curled up on her left side in bed. The physician diagnoses vaso-occlusive crisis.

Questions 8 to 10 refer to this situation.

8 A definitive diagnosis of sickle cell disease is based on which diagnostic results?

A. Complete blood count (CBC) and reticulocyte count
B. Bone marrow aspiration
C. Blood chemistry tests
D. Hemoglobin electrophoresis

9 Nursing care priorities for Vanessa include:

A. Providing I.V. fluids at 1½ times maintenance and administering pain medication, as prescribed
B. Administering antipyretic and pain medication, as prescribed
C. Monitoring vital signs every 15 minutes for 2 hours and administering pain medication, as prescribed
D. Establishing an I.V. line for packed red blood cell transfusions and obtaining a CBC, as prescribed

10 Vanessa exhibits a knowledge deficit about how she inherited sickle cell disease. The nurse should explain that the disease occurs when:

A. One parent has the disease
B. Neither parent has the disease
C. Both parents carry the sickle cell trait
D. One parent carries the sickle cell trait

Jeffrey, age 9, was diagnosed with hemophilia A shortly after birth, when he exhibited prolonged bleeding after circumcision. When learning to walk, he had frequent episodes of bleeding from the mouth; later, he began bleeding into muscles and joints. Now Jeffrey is on a home factor-replacement infusion program, and he and his parents determine when treatment is necessary for simple bleeding episodes.

Questions 11 and 12 refer to this situation.

11 An appropriate nursing measure for an infant or a young child with hemophilia is to:

A. Withhold all immunizations
B. Use a small-gauge needle and apply firm pressure after administering immunizations
C. Tell the parents to avoid routine dental visits for their child
D. Obtain a prescription for iron supplements

12 While walking to school, Jeffrey trips and falls on the sidewalk, scraping his knees and suffering a bruised and bleeding laceration of the forehead. His friends take him to the nurse's office. Which nursing action takes priority at this time?

A. Relieving his anxiety
B. Cleaning his knees
C. Cleaning his lacerated forehead
D. Assessing his level of consciousness

SITUATION

Tricia Graybill, age 6 months, is brought to the pediatrician for a routine well-child visit by her mother. The pediatrician orders a complete laboratory workup after physical examination reveals pallor and splenomegaly. Findings show a hematocrit of 15%, reticulocyte count of 4%, microcytosis, hypochromia, and target cell formation of red blood cells.

The pediatrician admits Tricia to the hospital and refers her to a pediatric hematologist. After a complete history and physical examination, the hematologist orders other laboratory tests, including hemoglobin electrophoresis. These tests confirm a diagnosis of beta-thalassemia major.

Questions 13 to 15 refer to this situation.

---

13 Tricia begins a blood transfusion program aimed at maintaining a hematocrit of approximately 30%. When considering the long-term effects of this treatment, the nurse is aware that blood transfusions:

A. Cannot prevent intercurrent infections
B. Cannot prevent continued delays in growth and development
C. Will improve Tricia's physical and psychological well-being, enabling her to participate in normal childhood activities
D. Cannot prevent onset of severe cardiomegaly by age 4

14 Tricia receives chelation therapy to eliminate excessive iron caused by repeated blood transfusions. What is the most effective way to administer deferoxamine mesylate (Desferal), the only drug indicated for iron removal?

A. By oral solution q.i.d.
B. By I.M. injection once a week
C. By subcutaneous infusion daily
D. By I.V. bolus with each blood transfusion

15 Tricia is at risk for life-threatening complications of iron overload. These complications include all of the following *except:*

A. Pericarditis, cardiac arrhythmias, and congestive heart failure
B. Central nervous system dysfunction
C. Hepatosplenomegaly
D. Endocrine dysfunction

SITUATION

Lynn Sabrick, age 18 months, is brought to the pediatrician's office for evaluation of petechiae on her back and shoulders and numerous ecchymoses extending down her arms and legs. Other than these symptoms, physical findings are normal, with no lymphadenopathy or hepatosplenomegaly. Except for an upper respiratory tract illness 2 weeks ago, she has been healthy; her immunizations are up to date.

To investigate the cause of petechiae and ecchymoses, the pediatrician orders a CBC, white blood cell (WBC) differential, and platelet count. Results show a WBC count of 6,200/mm³, hemoglobin level of 12.6 g/dl, hematocrit of 36.2%, platelet count of 12,000/mm³, neutrophil value of 40%, lymphocyte value of 48%, eosinophil value of 5%, basophil value of 1%, and monocyte value of 6%. Based on these findings, the pediatrician admits Lynn to the hospital and consults a pediatric hematologist to determine if she has idiopathic thrombocytopenic purpura (ITP).

Questions 16 and 17 refer to this situation.

16 To establish a diagnosis, the hematologist recommends that Lynn undergo bone marrow aspiration. The nurse knows that bone marrow aspiration is:

A. A painless procedure that takes about 5 minutes
B. Performed to rule out other causes of thrombocytopenia, such as leukemia
C. Performed to examine the bone marrow
D. Necessary only when the platelet count is below 20,000 mm^3

17 When planning Lynn's care, the nurse should consider that all of the following are true *except:*

A. Children with ITP rarely recover spontaneously
B. Children with ITP can be treated with corticosteroids
C. Children with ITP may be treated with I.V. gamma globulin
D. Children with ITP may be candidates for splenectomy if they have not maintained an adequate platelet count for 1 year

Answer sheet

A B C D
1 ○○○○
2 ○○○○
3 ○○○○
4 ○○○○
5 ○○○○
6 ○○○○
7 ○○○○
8 ○○○○
9 ○○○○
10 ○○○○
11 ○○○○
12 ○○○○
13 ○○○○
14 ○○○○
15 ○○○○
16 ○○○○
17 ○○○○

Answers and rationales

1 Correct answer—**C**

The normal hematocrit for a full-term neonate ranges from 55% to 65%. A hematocrit above 65% signals polycythemia.

2 Correct answer—**A**

Sickle cell disease, an inherited disorder, is characterized by an amino acid substitution in the beta-hemoglobin chain, referred to as *hemoglobin S* (Hgb S). Red blood cells (RBCs) lose their spherical shape and become sickle shaped, slowing blood flow and obstructing small vessels. In children ages 6 months to 2 years, vessel occlusion in short tubular bones typically causes painful swelling of the hands and feet. The spleen enlarges from congestion with sickled cells; the liver may enlarge from blood stasis. Other signs and symptoms of sickle cell disease in an infant include pallor and anemia, which result from the shortened life span of sickled cells. Leg ulcers are common in adolescents and adults. A fine macular rash may occur with skin conditions or drug allergies; it is not specific to sickle cell disease.

3 Correct answer—**D**

Breast-feeding—not bottle-feeding—is associated with an increased incidence of hyperbilirubinemia; however, the reason for this is not clear. An enclosed hemorrhage, such as cephalhematoma, and ABO blood incompatibility may cause an elevated serum bilirubin level from the increased rate of RBC hemolysis. Sepsis in a neonate may lead to vomiting and poor feeding, which may cause hyperbilirubinemia by increasing bilirubin absorption from the bowel.

4 Correct answer—**C**

The spleen is the main site of platelet destruction in children with idiopathic thrombocytopenic purpura (ITP) and the major organ involved in antibody synthesis and other host defense mechanisms. It also is crucial to antiplatelet antibody production. Therefore, after splenectomy the patient is at increased risk for bacterial infection and overwhelming sepsis. Administering a pneumococcal vaccine before surgery greatly decreases the risk of pneumococcal sepsis; however, septicemia may result from other organisms. After splenectomy, microorganisms may double in size within 20 to 40 minutes; therefore, parents should notify the physician when the child has a fever. Infection must be treated promptly, and prophylactic penicillin should be administered daily. The child should wear a medical identification tag that mentions she has had a splenectomy, which places her at increased risk for infection. For a child with a low platelet count, identification of ITP alerts caregivers in an emergency that the risk of hemorrhage is high.

5 Correct answer—A

Lead poisoning results from a toxic amount of lead in the body. Lead interferes with synthesis of heme, a substance needed for hemoglobin production. Iron-deficiency anemia results from a decrease in the body's iron supply, impaired iron absorption, or factors affecting hemoglobin synthesis. Impaired hemoglobin synthesis causes accumulation of hemoglobin precursors, such as erythrocyte protoporphyrin. Elevated levels of this precursor occur in both lead poisoning and iron-deficiency anemia. Hemophilia is a genetic bleeding disorder caused by deficiency of one of the factors necessary for coagulation. Anemia, thrombocytopenia, and leukopenia are common findings in aplastic anemia, which results from depressed bone marrow functioning. Idiopathic thrombocytic purpura manifests as thrombocytopenia and stems from excessive platelet destruction.

6 Correct answer—B

Gastric irritation, blackened stools, and darkened teeth are potential side effects of oral iron therapy. Pica may occur in children with iron-deficiency anemia but is not a side effect of iron therapy.

7 Correct answer—B

Iron supplements should be administered 1 hour before or 2 hours after meals with a citrus juice. Food and milk inhibit iron absorption; citrus juices enhance it.

8 Correct answer—D

Definitive diagnosis of sickle cell disease depends on hemoglobin electrophoresis, a test in which the various types of hemoglobin are separated and identified. The complete blood count and reticulocyte count help determine the severity of anemia and degree of bone marrow activity; these tests are useful in managing anemia associated with sickle cell disease. Bone marrow aspiration and blood chemistry tests are not used to diagnose sickle cell disease.

9 Correct answer—A

In a vaso-occlusive crisis, the hemoglobin S molecule is deoxygenated; it then polymerizes and forms long rods that distort RBCs, making them concave and sickle-shaped. Such RBCs cause increased blood viscosity and obstruct blood flow to the tissues; this in turn leads to ischemia and possible tissue necrosis. Providing I.V. fluids helps break up clumps of sickled cells, promoting tissue and RBC oxygenation; pain medication helps relax the child and decreases oxygen demands. Although an antipyretic commonly is administered to a patient with vaso-occlusive crisis, providing fluids takes a higher priority. Monitoring vital signs frequently, obtaining a complete blood count, and administering blood transfusions are appropriate actions for a child with splenic sequestration crisis, not vaso-occlusive crisis. In splenic sequestration crisis, a large volume of blood pools in the spleen, substantially reducing intravascular blood volume and ultimately causing shock.

10 Correct answer—C

Because sickle cell disease is an autosomal recessive disorder, both parents must carry the sickle cell trait for a child to inherit it. When both parents carry the trait, the child has a 25% chance of developing the disorder and a 50% chance of carrying the trait. If both parents have the disease, their children also will have it.

11 Correct answer—B

Children with hemophilia should be vaccinated according to a regular schedule. When immunizing a child with hemophilia, the nurse should use a small-gauge needle and apply pressure after the injection to prevent bleeding at the site. Regular dental care should be encouraged to prevent caries and gingivitis, a gum inflammation that predisposes the child to bleeding; use of a soft toothbrush helps avoid bleeding episodes. Iron supplementation is not indicated routinely for children with hemophilia.

12 Correct answer—D

Because intracranial hemorrhage is the most common cause of death in hemophiliac patients, any head injury should be investigated promptly; however, the nurse should keep in mind that signs and symptoms may be delayed. A patient who has a headache, nausea, vomiting, or decreased sensorium should be taken to the hospital. After determining that Jeffrey has not had an alteration in consciousness, the nurse should apply pressure and ice to the forehead laceration for at least 10 minutes to minimize bleeding. Reassuring Jeffrey that he did not sustain a serious injury can help relieve his anxiety, although this nursing action is not a priority. The forehead laceration and knee scrapes can be cleaned after other interventions are implemented.

13 Correct answer—C

Children with beta-thalassemia who receive RBC transfusions can grow and develop normally—at least until adolescence, when iron overload may impair growth and sexual development. For example, significant height retardation typically becomes evident by adolescence, and secondary sex characteristics may develop slowly or not at all. Children with beta-thalassemia may attend school and participate in normal childhood activities. Before RBC transfusions were available in treating beta-thalassemia, children with this disorder had significant problems with intercurrent infections, experienced delayed growth and development, and were prone to cardiomegaly.

14 Correct answer—C

The parenteral route—either continuous I.V. or subcutaneous infusion—currently is the most effective way to administer chelation therapy for iron overload. Deferoxamine mesylate usually is administered subcutaneously over an 8- to 10-hour period each day, 6 days a week, using a portable infusion pump. No oral chelating agents are available; I.M. administration of this agent is less effective than subcutaneous administration.

15 Correct answer—B

Iron overload does not affect the central nervous system. Excess iron is stored in various body tissues, including the heart, liver, spleen, gallbladder, and pancreas. Such an excess causes tissue fibrosis through an unknown mechanism. Cardiac tissue fibrosis leads to arrhythmias and congestive heart failure; fibrosis of the spleen and liver leads to splenomegaly and hepatomegaly, respectively. Endocrine glands are extremely sensitive to iron levels and may become dysfunctional even from small amounts of stored iron; pancreatic dysfunction may cause diabetes mellitus.

16 Correct answer—B

The bone marrow produces RBCs, white blood cells, and platelets. Bone marrow aspiration is performed to assess bone marrow function and to rule out other causes of thrombocytopenia, such as leukemia. In a patient with ITP, bone marrow aspirate usually reveals normocellular tissue with an increased number of megakaryocytes (platelet precursors). The procedure is painful; the child may need to be restrained or sedated while the specimen is obtained.

17 Correct answer—A

Up to 95% of children with ITP recover spontaneously within 4 months. When planning care for Lynn, the nurse should consider her platelet count, age, and activity level. Platelet count reflects the risk of bleeding. Age is a consideration because of the potential complications of corticosteroid therapy (such as growth retardation) and splenectomy (such as infection). Active children are at increased risk for hemorrhage when the platelet count is low. Active children and those who injure themselves frequently may benefit from aggressive therapy; less active children can be managed by close monitoring of the platelet count.

The physician may choose to observe the child, obtain frequent platelet counts, or treat the condition with corticosteroids or I.V. gamma globulin (IVGG). Corticosteroids are administered to children at high risk for bleeding (as indicated by a platelet count below 30,000 mm^3). These drugs may inhibit removal of sensitized platelets by the reticuloendothelial system; IVGG may stimulate platelet production.

The spleen contains a large amount of reticuloendothelial cells, which remove blood elements and carry out phagocytosis of particulate matter. Splenectomy is considered in cases of life-threatening hemorrhage or menorrhagia that does not respond to hormone treatment. Older children who do not respond to corticosteroids or IVGG also may be candidates for splenectomy to inhibit excessive platelet destruction caused by ITP.

CHAPTER 16

Comprehensive Examination

Questions

1 An infant's birth weight should triple by which age?

  A. 4 months
  B. 6 months
  C. 9 months
  D. 12 months

2 Hydrocephalus is a condition characterized by:

  A. A defect in the growth of the brain
  B. An imbalance in the production and absorption of cerebrospinal fluid (CSF)
  C. Protrusion of meninges and CSF in a saclike cyst
  D. Herniation of the brain and meninges through a defect in the skull

3 Blood pressure that varies among extremities is a common finding in children with:

  A. Aortic stenosis
  B. Coarctation of the aorta
  C. Patent ductus arteriosus
  D. Atrial septal defect

4 Which congenital cardiac anomaly is associated with tetralogy of Fallot (TOF)?

  A. Origination of the aorta from the right ventricle and origination of the pulmonary artery from the left ventricle
  B. A hole in the ventricular septum allowing communication between the ventricles
  C. Pulmonary stenosis, right ventricular hypertrophy, ventricular septal defect, and dextroposition of the aorta
  D. Narrowing of the aorta, restricting left ventricular outflow

5 The best time to perform chest physiotherapy on a child is:

  A. After aerosol therapy, in conjunction with breathing exercises
  B. Immediately after meals
  C. Once in the morning and once in the evening
  D. When the child has a pulmonary infection

6 Which statement about cystic fibrosis is *true?*

A. It is a disorder involving excess mucus production in the lungs and digestive tract
B. It causes obstruction of the bronchi and bronchioles from bronchospasm
C. It causes allergic reactions to food, dust, or other substances, such as smoke or pollens
D. It is characterized by polyps in the respiratory tract that impede breathing

7 A lumbosacral meningomyelocele is removed at birth to:

A. Improve circulation in the lower extremities
B. Reverse nerve damage to the spinal cord
C. Increase the chance for a successful shunting procedure
D. Decrease the risk of secondary meningitis

8 When caring for a child with laryngotracheobronchitis (croup), the nurse's main concern is to:

A. Prevent bronchial spasm
B. Detect wheezing
C. Promote drainage of lung secretions
D. Maintain a patent airway

9 An appropriate nursing action for a neonate receiving phototherapy for hyperbilirubinemia is to:

A. Turn the neonate frequently
B. Administer frequent feedings
C. Monitor fluid intake and output
D. All of the above

10 Finger clubbing in an infant is caused by:

A. Acidosis
B. Chronic tissue hypoxia
C. Edema
D. Polycythemia

11 Discharge planning for the parents of a child with TOF should include all of the following *except:*

A. Demonstrating the knee-to-chest position
B. Instructing them to increase the child's fluid intake during hot weather and periods of fever, vomiting, or diarrhea
C. Instructing them to limit the child's activity level
D. Instructing them to provide the child with small, frequent feedings

12 Before cardiac catheterization, the nurse should prepare a pediatric patient for which procedure?

A. Administration of a dextrose I.V. solution to prevent hypoglycemia
B. Electroencephalography to detect arrhythmias
C. Administration of general anesthesia during the invasive procedure
D. Administration of supplemental oxygen

13 Which statement about seizures in a child is *not* true?

A. If the child has aspirated vomitus, the caregiver should seek medical attention as soon as possible
B. To prevent injury, the caregiver should restrain the child's arms and legs
C. To prevent injury, the child should be turned on the side and nothing should be forced into the mouth
D. The caregiver should note the time that the seizure began and ended as well as events that preceded and immediately followed it

14 Which osmotic diuretic commonly is administered to reduce increased intracranial pressure (ICP)?

A. Mannitol (Osmitrol)
B. Hydrochlorothiazide (Aprozide)
C. Furosemide (Lasix)
D. Diphenhydramine (Benadryl)

15 Nursing care for a child with increased ICP includes:

A. Elevating the head of the bed 60 degrees
B. Avoiding neck vein compression
C. Performing vigorous range-of-motion exercises
D. Performing chest percussion

16 Which activity promotes cognitive development in a school-age child (ages 6 to 12)?

A. Playing kickball
B. Playing Scrabble
C. Painting by numbers
D. Building a tree fort

17 The most appropriate way for a caregiver to provide visual stimulation to a 1-month-old infant is to:

A. Hold the infant face to face at a distance of 8″ to 10″ (20 to 25 cm)
B. Hang a mobile about 12″ (30 cm) above the infant's crib
C. Hold the infant on the lap while watching television
D. Manipulate a puppet about 6″ (15 cm) in front of the infant

18 For a school-age child who is immobilized on the pediatric unit, which nursing action would thwart the child's ability to develop and master skills?

A. Praising the child for all appropriate activities
B. Displaying the child's art work on the unit even if he denies permission to do so
C. Encouraging the child to engage in group play
D. Encouraging the child to engage in bedside activities that he can accomplish alone

19 A couple with a child who has a homozygous recessive trait are unaffected by the trait themselves. The probability that their second child will have the same trait is:

A. 25%
B. 50%
C. 75%
D. 100%

20 Which complication is most common in neonates with necrotizing enterocolitis?

A. Hydrocephalus
B. Pneumothorax
C. Cholecystitis
D. Intestinal perforation

21 The stools of a healthy, exclusively breast-fed 2-week-old neonate typically are:

A. Greenish brown and semisolid, occurring once or twice a day
B. Easy to pass but irritating to the neonate's sensitive skin
C. Yellowish, formed, and sweet-smelling
D. Yellowish and loose or watery, occurring at nearly every feeding

22 A neonate demonstrates the tonic neck reflex by:

A. Extending the leg on the side to which the head is turned
B. Flexing the leg on the side to which the head is turned
C. Extending the leg on the side opposite to which the head is turned
D. Abducting the leg on the side opposite to which the head is turned

23 When assessing a school-age child or adolescent, the nurse should screen for which musculoskeletal deviation?

A. Hip dysplasia
B. Scoliosis
C. Osteogenesis imperfecta
D. All of the above

24 Which nursing action would best help a child to relax during an abdominal examination?

A. Touching the child with cool hands
B. Positioning the child with hips flexed and knees bent
C. Palpating tender areas first
D. Performing the examination without warning the child what to expect

25 Primary amenorrhea is defined as menarche delayed after age:

A. 10
B. 12
C. 15
D. 17

26 When assessing a child who claims to have been sexually abused, the nurse should keep in mind that:

A. Children have vivid imaginations and sometimes make up situations involving sexual activities
B. Children sometimes lie about sexual abuse to hide their masturbatory activities
C. Children seldom lie about sexual abuse
D. Children sometimes lie about sexual abuse as a way of expressing jealousy over parental relationships

27 When teaching an adolescent about oral contraceptives, the nurse should include all of the following points *except:*

A. Dosage schedule
B. Side effects
C. Need for regular medical checkups
D. Need to reduce caloric intake to avoid weight gain

28 Which statement about prenatal counseling for an adolescent patient is *true?*

A. Individual counseling is best because it allows for personalized teaching
B. Peer group acceptance is imperative if the adolescent is to accept her pregnancy
C. Individual counseling is optimal because it provides an adult role model
D. Group counseling is most effective if the adolescent participants are in the same trimester of pregnancy

29 A child with cleft palate is at risk for hearing problems because of:

A. An immature acoustic nerve
B. Recurrent otitis media
C. Poor bone conduction
D. Congenital ear anomalies

30 Immediately after cleft palate repair, an infant should be placed in which position?

A. Right side-lying
B. Semi-Fowler's
C. Prone
D. Left side-lying

31 The nurse should encourage the parents of a child with cleft palate to promote the child's speech development by:

A. Correcting his speech
B. Playing speaking games
C. Reading him stories
D. Using baby talk

32 Which finding suggests esophagitis in a child with gastroesophageal reflux?

A. Rattling cough
B. Apnea
C. Pallor
D. Occult blood in the stool

33 Esophageal atresia may lead to respiratory distress. Which of the following is *not* a sign of respiratory distress in a neonate?

A. Tachycardia
B. Bradycardia
C. Nasal flaring
D. Chest retractions

34 Which data would support the suspicion of anorexia nervosa in a girl age 13 who is below the 5th percentile for her weight?

A. She frequently looks at her body in the mirror, has lost 10 lb (4.5 kg) during the last 2 months, eats only small helpings of food, and binges secretly
B. She has lost 30 lb (13.6 kg) during the past year and always skips breakfast
C. She dislikes her body, reports an intense interest in preparing and serving food but claims to have no appetite, has had a marked weight loss, and is preoccupied with exercising
D. She binges, then fasts; has frequent weight fluctuations; and dislikes shopping for clothes because she says everything makes her look fat

35 When an adolescent has signs and symptoms of anorexia nervosa, the most appropriate initial nursing intervention is to:

A. Talk to her about life stresses
B. Teach her parents how to prepare nutritious meals and snacks
C. Ask her to keep a food diary and weigh her every 2 weeks
D. Encourage her parents to seek help from a professional who specializes in eating disorders

36 Decorticate posturing is characterized by:

A. Adduction of the arms at the shoulders
B. Abduction of the arms at the shoulders
C. Extension of the wrists
D. Flexion of the legs at the knees

37 The most common cause of hyperbilirubinemia in a full-term neonate is:

A. Polycythemia
B. Biliary atresia
C. Enzyme deficiencies
D. Immature liver function

38 During the first 24 hours after a child has undergone tonsillectomy or adenoidectomy, the nurse should observe the child closely for:

A. Frequent swallowing
B. Refusal to eat
C. Complaint of headache
D. Respiratory stridor

39 When a child can tolerate cool water after tonsillectomy or adenoidectomy, the nurse can begin offering:

A. Cold milk
B. Apple juice
C. Grape or cherry soda
D. Fruit juice

40 Laboratory and radiographic evaluation for Hodgkin's disease includes all of the following tests *except:*

A. Barium enema
B. Erythrocyte sedimentation rate
C. Gallium scan
D. Chest X-ray

41 Which statement about proper care for a central venous line in a pediatric patient is *true?*

A. A heparin solution should never be used to keep the central line patent
B. A normal saline flush is sufficient to prevent the central line from clotting
C. A full-strength heparin solution should be used to prevent the central line from clotting
D. A reduced-strength heparin solution should be used to prevent the central line from clotting

42 The most common cause of hyperbilirubinemia in a full-term neonate is:

A. Polycythemia
B. Biliary atresia
C. Enzyme deficiencies
D. Immature liver function

43 Calcium levels are highest in which food?

A. Broccoli
B. Prunes
C. Nuts
D. Papaya

44 Which question effectively elicits information about a caregiver's knowledge of toilet training?

A. "Have you had any experience with toilet training?"
B. "Has your child shown any interest in toilet training?"
C. "What do you know about toilet training?"
D. "Why do you want to toilet train your child?"

45 During which activity can the nurse best assess infant-caregiver interaction?

A. Sleeping
B. Feeding
C. Playing
D. Rocking

46 In pubescent boys, pubic hair formation begins at the base of the:

A. Scrotum
B. Penis
C. Scrotum and penis
D. Inguinal lymph glands

47 What is the correct hand placement for cardiac compression in an infant?

A. Above the nipple line
B. At the nipple line
C. One finger-width below the nipple line
D. At the xiphoid

48 What is the most common reason for abdominal surgery in a child over age 2?

A. Appendicitis
B. Phimosis
C. Inguinal hernia
D. Hydrocele

49 Which signs and symptoms commonly manifest when a child develops diabetes mellitus?

A. Polyuria, polydipsia, and weight loss
B. Abnormally low urine specific gravity
C. Nocturnal enuresis or nocturia
D. Both A and C

50 Which information is most important when assessing a child with a suspected respiratory tract infection?

A. Hydration status
B. School activity
C. Immunization reports
D. Surrounding vegetation

51 For lumbar puncture, an infant should be placed in:

A. An arched, side-lying position with the neck flexed onto the chest
B. An arched, side-lying position that avoids flexion of the neck onto the chest
C. A mummy restraint
D. A prone position with the head over the edge of the table or bed

---

SITUATION

Darlene Collingwood, age 6 months, is brought to the well-child clinic for a routine immunization by her mother. Mrs. Collingwood tells the physician that Darlene has difficulty sucking and swallowing, vomits frequently, is irritable, and seems stiff when held. Darlene weighed 4 lb (1,800 g) when born at 28 weeks' gestation. After further evaluation, the physician suspects cerebral palsy.

Questions 52 and 53 refer to this situation.

52 When performing physical assessment of an infant with suspected cerebral palsy, the nurse should pay particular attention to all of the following findings *except:*

A. Vision, hearing, and speech problems
B. Persistence of primitive reflexes
C. Impaired arm or leg movement
D. Hemangioma on the buttocks

53 After testing and further evaluation, Darlene is diagnosed with the spastic quadriplegia form of cerebral palsy. Patients with this condition typically exhibit:

A. A combination of symptoms
B. A poor sense of balance and depth perception
C. Tense, contracted muscles
D. Constant uncontrolled movements

Mrs. Collingwood brings Darlene, now age 5, to the clinic for a routine checkup.

Questions 54 to 57 continue the preceding situation.

54 To elicit appropriate information about Darlene's gross motor development, the nurse should ask Mrs. Collingwood which question?

A. "Does she have any hearing problems?"
B. "Does she have any visual problems?"
C. "Does she hop and run?"
D. "Can she identify any colors?"

55 Which behavior by Mrs. Collingwood would lead the nurse to suspect that she has not accepted her daughter's diagnosis?

A. She refuses to place the child in a special education program
B. She recognizes her child's defects but tries to focus on her as whole
C. She recognizes when Darlene becomes fatigued during therapy
D. She participates in a parental support group

56 Which assessment data would lead the nurse to formulate a nursing diagnosis of *Feeding self-care deficit related to neuromuscular impairment* for Darlene?

A. Inaccurate interpretation of environmental stimuli
B. Inability to bring food from plate to mouth
C. Swallowing only liquid foods
D. Dislike of many foods

57 Which nursing intervention most effectively would promote a positive self-image in Darlene?

A. Discussing with family members the importance of accepting Darlene
B. Encouraging Darlene to interact socially with her peers
C. Noting signs of grieving or depression in Darlene
D. Discouraging Darlene from discussing her disability

SITUATION

Lonnie, age 5, is admitted to the pediatric unit with a diagnosis of acute lymphoblastic leukemia. She has begun induction chemotherapy and 2 days ago received transfusions of packed red blood cells and platelets to correct anemia and thrombocytopenia. Today, her laboratory values are: white blood cell count, 1,600 mm³; hemoglobin level, 10 g/dl; hematocrit, 28.2%; platelet count, 152,000 mm³; segmented neutrophil count, 50%; lymphocyte count, 38%; monocyte count, 10%; and eosinophil count, 2%. On the 28th day of therapy, results of Lonnie's bone marrow aspiration indicate that she is in remission.

Questions 58 to 61 refer to this situation.

58 At this time, the greatest threat to Lonnie's health is:

A. Anemia
B. Thrombocytopenia
C. Infection
D. Stroke

59 The nurse begins teaching Lonnie and her family ways to prevent complications. Which is the best general guideline for them to follow?

A. If Lonnie's absolute neutrophil count is low, she should avoid crowds; if her platelet count is low, she should avoid contact sports and activities that could cause injury
B. If Lonnie's absolute neutrophil count is low, she should avoid school and sports or physical activities
C. If Lonnie's absolute neutrophil count is low, she should wear a mask and wash her hands frequently
D. Lonnie should keep immunizations current and avoid strenuous physical activity

60 The nurse determines that Lonnie needs help in coping with her diagnosis and treatment. All of the following are appropriate nursing actions *except:*

A. Allowing her to play with a toy medical kit
B. Discussing the disease with her and explaining how chemotherapeutic drugs work
C. Allowing her to choose which leg will receive the injection
D. Reassuring her that she has no reason to fear her treatment

61 Lonnie's mother asks why her daughter's treatment must continue for 2½ years. The nurse's best response would be:

A. "That's the way her protocol is designed"
B. "Research shows that this duration is best for preventing a relapse"
C. "Although Lonnie is in remission, leukemic cells may be hiding in her body. We have to be sure to destroy as many of them as possible"
D. "Lonnie is at high risk for relapse because of the type of leukemia she has"

SITUATION

Julie, age 17, visits the physician complaining of frequent weight fluctuations, uncontrolled eating binges, and dependence on laxatives. A cheerleader with a 3.8 grade point average, she describes herself as a perfectionist. Despite her achievements, Julie reports feeling "fat and stupid." She is 5'6" (167.6 cm) tall and weighs 136 lb (61.7 kg). The physician diagnoses bulimia.

Questions 62 to 64 refer to this situation.

62 Early identification of an eating disorder improves the outlook for recovery. Which assessment area is *least* helpful in identifying an eating disorder?

A. Body image
B. Family dynamics
C. Personality structure and related behaviors
D. Athletic achievements

63 Julie is at risk for which potentially dangerous condition?

A. Diabetes
B. Electrolyte imbalance
C. Diarrhea
D. Anemia

64 Which trait is most characteristic in a patient with bulimia?

A. Low self-esteem
B. Aggression
C. Assertiveness
D. Creativity

SITUATION

David, age 18 months, is small and pale, with thin arms and legs and a distended abdomen. His mother reports that he has been slow to gain weight and has had frequent respiratory tract infections, some of which required hospitalization for pneumonia. He now has another infection and has been admitted to the hospital for diagnostic tests for cystic fibrosis.

Questions 65 and 66 refer to this situation.

65 Which assessment finding would the nurse expect in a child with cystic fibrosis?

A. Decreased sweat electrolyte levels
B. Presence of pancreatic enzymes
C. Family history of cystic fibrosis
D. Increased fat absorption

66 David is diagnosed with cystic fibrosis. Dietary planning for him should include all of the following *except:*

A. Replacement of pancreatic enzymes
B. Additional use of salt during hot weather
C. Adherence to a fat-free diet
D. Ingestion of a water-miscible daily multivitamin

SITUATION

Krystal, a full-term neonate, is diagnosed with meconium aspiration syndrome necessitating oxygen therapy. She tests positive for phenylketonuria (PKU).

Questions 67 and 68 refer to this situation.

67 PKU is an inherited disorder characterized by inability to:

A. Retain phenylalanine
B. Decrease myelinization
C. Convert phenylalanine to tyrosine
D. Conjugate phenylalanine in the liver

68 All of the following statements about PKU are true *except:*

A. Irritability and vomiting are signs of PKU in neonates
B. Eczema is common in infants with PKU
C. The urine of neonates with PKU may have a musty (mousy) smell
D. At age 1 to 2 months, an infant with PKU may have a large, soft anterior fontanel and a large tongue

SITUATION

Grace, age 9, is admitted to the pediatric unit with status asthmaticus. The physician orders an aminophylline drip (1 mg/ml) to be infused at 28 ml/hour; I.V. dextrose 10% in water at 10 ml/hour; and I.V. hydrocortisone, 18 mg every 4 hours.

Questions 69 to 71 refer to this situation.

69 All of the following are signs or symptoms of aminophylline toxicity *except:*

A. Restlessness or nervousness
B. Slightly decreased heart rate
C. Twitching or seizures
D. Hyperactive reflexes

70 Priorities for a child with asthma include:

A. Attending school regularly, avoiding the need for emergency medical care, and preventing upper respiratory tract infections
B. Attending school regularly, avoiding hospitalization, participating in activities, and having a normal family life
C. Participating in sports, avoiding situations that trigger asthma attacks, and being weaned from medication
D. Attending school regularly, participating in sports, and avoiding asthma attacks

71 Grace is discharged from the hospital and placed on a home medication regimen. She takes her medications regularly as directed. In case of an asthma attack, she should be instructed to:

A. Take another dose of medication and rest
B. Rest and do breathing exercises
C. Remain calm, drink plenty of tepid fluids, use her metered-dose inhaler as instructed, and seek medical attention if the attack does not subside within a reasonable time
D. Do breathing exercises, use her metered-dose inhaler, and go to the nearest emergency department immediately

SITUATION

Alex, born 4 hours ago, is being maintained under a radiant heater in the neonatal nursery.

Questions 72 to 76 refer to this situation.

72 Which signs in Alex would lead the nurse to suspect that he has a tracheoesophageal fistula (TEF)?

A. Projectile vomiting and increased bowel sounds
B. Abdominal distention and visible peristalsis
C. Decreased respiratory secretions and diminished breath sounds
D. Excessive oral mucus and choking during feeding

73 Which intervention is appropriate when the nurse suspects TEF in a neonate?

A. Initiating oral feedings of dextrose in water
B. Initiating nasogastric tube feedings of dextrose in water, as ordered
C. Withholding all oral feedings
D. Feeding the neonate a bottle in an upright position

74 To prevent aspiration, the nurse should place Alex in which position?

A. Trendelenburg
B. Supine with the head of the crib elevated 30 to 45 degrees
C. Right lateral decubitus
D. Prone with the head of the crib elevated 60 to 90 degrees

75 Which equipment should the nurse keep on hand when caring for Alex?

A. Bulb syringe
B. Tongue blade and artificial airway
C. Endotracheal suctioning device
D. Tracheostomy set

76 TEF is associated with which complication?

A. Necrotizing enterocolitis
B. Bronchopulmonary dysplasia
C. Chemical pneumonitis
D. Anorectal anomaly

SITUATION

Maria, age 2, is admitted to the hospital with pneumonia. Mrs. Price, her grandmother, tells the nurse that Maria has had a temperature of 102° F (38.9° C) with coughing and irritability for the past 2 days. She also reports that Maria has been hospitalized five times for previous infections and failure to thrive. Her mother, an I.V. drug abuser with acquired immunodeficiency syndrome (AIDS), frequently leaves Maria with Mrs. Price.

Questions 77 to 93 refer to this situation.

77 Because of Maria's medical history and her mother's drug abuse and AIDS diagnosis, the physician most likely will order which tests to determine whether Maria carries antibodies to the AIDS virus?

A. Wasserman and Western blot
B. Enzyme-linked immunosorbent assay (ELISA) and Western blot
C. ELISA and Wasserman
D. Wasserman and AZT

78 Besides a positive blood test, which criteria are used to diagnose AIDS in a child?

A. Presence of risk factors, an opportunistic infection, and no other diagnosed immune disease
B. Presence of risk factors, a diagnosed immune disease, and multiple infections
C. Household contact with human immunodeficiency virus (HIV), an opportunistic infection, and a diagnosed immune disease
D. Household contact with HIV, multiple infections, and no other diagnosed immune disease

79 Maria is diagnosed with AIDS. After obtaining a detailed history, the nurse must perform a thorough physical assessment to determine the child's:

A. Baseline data and presence of abnormalities
B. Baseline data and genetic predisposition
C. Genetic predisposition and presence of abnormalities
D. Genetic and social predisposition to AIDS

80 Maria undergoes a developmental assessment. What is the rationale for performing this assessment?

A. Children with AIDS typically develop slowly
B. Children with AIDS typically have accelerated development
C. Children with AIDS typically regress physically but not psychosocially
D. None of the above

81 Sandra Lawson, a new nurse at the hospital, is reluctant to care for Maria because of Maria's diagnosis of AIDS. The nurse-manager should:

A. Support Sandra's decision to refuse to care for Maria, which is in accordance with the Code for Nurses
B. Assign Sandra to another unit
C. Deny Sandra's right to refuse to care for Maria
D. Educate and counsel Sandra about AIDS

82 Maria is having trouble gaining weight. Which action should the nurse take to determine her dietary intake?

A. Measure her weight daily
B. Check her birth weight
C. Count her daily caloric intake
D. Measure her fluid intake and output

83 Maria's physician decides to perform bronchoscopy. In this case, the main purpose of bronchoscopy is to:

A. Remove a mucus plug
B. Assess the extent of pneumonia
C. Perform bronchial lavage
D. Determine the type of pneumonia

84 Which precautions must the nurse take when caring for Maria?

A. Respiratory precautions
B. Enteric precautions
C. Blood precautions
D. Universal precautions

85 Which nursing diagnosis applies to Maria?

A. Diarrhea related to failure to thrive
B. Impaired gas exchange related to respiratory infection
C. Impaired skin integrity related to failure to thrive
D. Impaired physical mobility related to the diagnosis of AIDS

86 The physician orders total parenteral nutrition for Maria. The purpose of this therapy is to:

A. Increase her fluid intake
B. Decrease the risk of infection
C. Increase her caloric intake
D. Provide a means for administering parenteral medications

87 The nurse should incorporate structural play into Maria's daily routine. Which toys are appropriate for her?

A. Blocks
B. Beads to string
C. Puzzles
D. Stuffed animals

88 Maria is receiving I.V. antibiotics. Which side effect is most common with these drugs?

A. Decreased appetite
B. Diarrhea
C. Stomach pain
D. Vomiting

89 When preparing Maria for discharge, an appropriate nursing measure would be to:

A. Arrange for her outpatient medication regimen
B. Arrange for her transportation home
C. Refer her for hospice care
D. Observe her primary caregiver

90 Mrs. Price expresses fear that other family members will contract AIDS from Maria. The nurse should address this concern by:

A. Planning a home assessment visit to observe how the family lives
B. Arranging a meeting with the family of another AIDS patient
C. Encouraging family involvement in a support group for AIDS patients
D. Educating the family about AIDS transmission modes

91 Maria's compromised immune system predisposes her to multiple infections. To reduce the risk of infection, the nurse should instruct her caregiver to:

A. Administer vitamin and mineral supplements
B. Schedule regular clinic visits
C. Provide a balanced diet
D. Keep her away from people with infections

92 Two weeks after Maria is discharged from the hospital, Mrs. Price calls the clinic to report that her granddaughter has a temperature of 101° F (38.3° C), chills, coughing, and wheezing. Which action should the nurse recommend?

A. Giving the child 80 mg of acetaminophen (Tylenol) and performing chest percussion
B. Giving the child 80 mg of acetaminophen and placing her in a humidified room
C. Bringing the child to the clinic for further evaluation
D. Giving the child a sponge bath and forcing fluids

93 Mrs. Price becomes overprotective and restricts Maria from playing with other children. What should the nurse tell her regarding these actions?

A. Her actions are appropriate to protect Maria from injury
B. Her actions are inappropriate because Maria needs to maintain a normal life-style
C. Her actions are appropriate because Maria should not play with other children
D. Her actions are appropriate ways of protecting Maria from infection

---

SITUATION

Susie McCann, age 6 months, is brought to the emergency department with a temperature of 105° F (40.5° C), vomiting, and irritability. During the nursing assessment, Susie has a seizure. The physician orders lumbar puncture followed by I.V. therapy, then admits Susie to the pediatric unit for further testing to rule out meningitis.

Questions 94 to 96 refer to this situation.

94 Which assessment finding in Susie would be most significant?

A. Kernig's sign
B. Bulging fontanels
C. Photophobia
D. Second heart sound (S_2)

95 Susie is kept in respiratory isolation in the pediatric unit. The nurse explains to Mrs. McCann the reason for isolation. Which statement by Mrs. McCann would indicate that this teaching was effective?

A. "I must put on a mask and gown and wash my hands before visiting Susie"
B. "I must wear gloves when touching Susie's diapers"
C. "Because Susie's resistance is low, I must wear a mask and gown when visiting and keep anyone with a cold out of the room"
D. "I know meningitis can be fatal, so I will put on a mask, gown, and gloves and wash my hands before visiting Susie"

96 Susie's order for I.V. fluids is less than her body requirements because the physician is attempting to prevent:

A. Circulatory overload
B. Electrolyte imbalance
C. Kidney failure
D. Cerebral edema

SITUATION

Christopher, an 8-year-old hemophiliac patient, has been coming to the clinic for 6 years. During the past year, he has had multiple infections, including two bouts of pneumonia requiring hospitalization. During today's clinic visit, the physician informs his parents that Christopher has tested positive for HIV. The positive test result and his medical history indicate that Christopher has AIDS.

Questions 97 to 100 refer to this situation.

97 Which statement is true when a patient tests positive for HIV?

A. The patient has developed an immunity to HIV
B. The patient has developed antibodies to HIV
C. The patient has a diagnosis of AIDS-related complex
D. The patient has a diagnosis of HIV

98 The nurse must assess how much Christopher's parents know about AIDS because:

A. Other family members are at high risk for the disease
B. AIDS is transmitted easily through casual contact
C. AIDS is a common complication of hemophilia
D. Many misconceptions exist about AIDS

99 Christopher has a nosebleed at school. How should the teacher and school nurse handle this problem?

A. They should use gauze pads and ice to control the bleeding
B. They should allow the bleeding to stop spontaneously
C. They should attempt to control the bleeding while wearing gloves
D. They should notify Christopher's parents and physician

100 Which solution is recommended for disinfecting surfaces contaminated by HIV-infected body fluids?

A. 1 part ammonia to 10 parts water
B. 1 part chlorine bleach to 10 parts water
C. 1 part alcohol to 10 parts water
D. 1 part detergent to 10 parts water

Answer sheet

A B C D	A B C D	A B C D	A B C D
1 ○○○○	31 ○○○○	61 ○○○○	91 ○○○○
2 ○○○○	32 ○○○○	62 ○○○○	92 ○○○○
3 ○○○○	33 ○○○○	63 ○○○○	93 ○○○○
4 ○○○○	34 ○○○○	64 ○○○○	94 ○○○○
5 ○○○○	35 ○○○○	65 ○○○○	95 ○○○○
6 ○○○○	36 ○○○○	66 ○○○○	96 ○○○○
7 ○○○○	37 ○○○○	67 ○○○○	97 ○○○○
8 ○○○○	38 ○○○○	68 ○○○○	98 ○○○○
9 ○○○○	39 ○○○○	69 ○○○○	99 ○○○○
10 ○○○○	40 ○○○○	70 ○○○○	100 ○○○○
11 ○○○○	41 ○○○○	71 ○○○○	
12 ○○○○	42 ○○○○	72 ○○○○	
13 ○○○○	43 ○○○○	73 ○○○○	
14 ○○○○	44 ○○○○	74 ○○○○	
15 ○○○○	45 ○○○○	75 ○○○○	
16 ○○○○	46 ○○○○	76 ○○○○	
17 ○○○○	47 ○○○○	77 ○○○○	
18 ○○○○	48 ○○○○	78 ○○○○	
19 ○○○○	49 ○○○○	79 ○○○○	
20 ○○○○	50 ○○○○	80 ○○○○	
21 ○○○○	51 ○○○○	81 ○○○○	
22 ○○○○	52 ○○○○	82 ○○○○	
23 ○○○○	53 ○○○○	83 ○○○○	
24 ○○○○	54 ○○○○	84 ○○○○	
25 ○○○○	55 ○○○○	85 ○○○○	
26 ○○○○	56 ○○○○	86 ○○○○	
27 ○○○○	57 ○○○○	87 ○○○○	
28 ○○○○	58 ○○○○	88 ○○○○	
29 ○○○○	59 ○○○○	89 ○○○○	
30 ○○○○	60 ○○○○	90 ○○○○	

Answers and rationales

1 Correct answer—**D**

Birth weight typically doubles by 6 months, triples by 12 months, and quadruples by 30 months.

2 Correct answer—**B**

Hydrocephalus is a condition characterized by an imbalance in the production and absorption of cerebrospinal fluid (CSF). Microcephaly is a defect in the growth of the brain. Meningocele is a saclike protrusion of meninges and CSF. Encephalocele is a herniation of the brain and meninges through a defect in the skull.

3 Correct answer—**B**

A child with coarctation of the aorta—congenital narrowing of the aorta—has bounding pulses and high blood pressure in areas of the body receiving blood from vessels proximal to the defect. A child with patent ductus arteriosus typically has a wide pulse pressure resulting from a low diastolic pressure caused by the shunting of blood. Aortic stenosis is characterized by a systolic murmur. Atrial septal defect is characterized by a harsh systolic murmur.

4 Correct answer—**C**

Tetralogy of Fallot (TOF) is characterized by four defects—pulmonary stenosis, right ventricular hypertrophy, ventricular septal defect, and dextroposition of the aorta. TOF is the most common cyanotic heart defect in children. Origination of the aorta from the right ventricle and origination of the pulmonary artery from the left ventricle characterizes transposition of the great vessels. A hole in the ventricular septum characterizes ventricular septal defect. Narrowing of the aorta occurs in aortic stenosis.

5 Correct answer—**A**

Chest physiotherapy (CPT) and breathing exercises help maintain effective drainage of bronchial secretions. In the hospital, CPT usually is performed after aerosol therapy; aerosol and mist therapy dilate the bronchial tree, maximizing the effects of treatment. CPT should be delayed for at least 1 hour after meals because of the risk of vomiting. Usually, it is performed three to four times a day; twice a day is insufficient. CPT should be performed as a preventive measure before a child develops a pulmonary infection.

6 Correct answer—**A**

In cystic fibrosis, exocrine (mucus-producing) glands release excessive amounts of extremely viscous mucus, which blocks secretion of pancreatic enzymes needed for digestion and interferes with nutrient absorption in the intestine. Mucus accumulation also obstructs airway passages in the lungs and causes patches of atelectasis and generalized emphysema. Pulmonary involvement is progressive and severe. Bronchial and bronchiolar obstruction result from excessive mucus, not bronchospasm. Cystic fibrosis appears to be mediated by an inherited biochemical deviation (possibly an enzyme); it is not an allergic response. Nasal polyps may develop in children with cystic fibrosis but are not the main cause of impeded breathing.

7 Correct answer—**D**

The meningomyelocele sac is removed as soon as possible to prevent meningitis, which may result from entry of bacteria into the central nervous system (CNS) through an opening in the sac. Surgery cannot reverse nerve damage occurring at birth, nor does it have a bearing on circulation or successful shunt placement.

8 Correct answer—**D**

Laryngotracheobronchitis—inflammation of the larynx, trachea, and bronchi with subglottic edema—requires a patent airway to ensure proper oxygenation. Accumulated lung secretions, bronchial spasms, and wheezing are not associated with this disorder.

9 Correct answer—**D**

Phototherapy, in which the neonate is exposed to special blue or cool white lights, reduces the serum bilirubin level by photoisomerizing bilirubin to nontoxic isomers in the extravascular space. These isomers diffuse into the blood and bind to albumin; from here, they are transported to the liver and excreted by the bowel. For phototherapy, the neonate is placed nude under the lights wearing protective eye and genital coverings. The nurse must turn the neonate to allow exposure of all skin surfaces. Frequent feedings promote hydration and caloric intake, increasing bowel motility and reducing bilirubin resorption from the bowel. Phototherapy may cause dehydration from insensible fluid loss and fluid loss from the gastrointestinal (GI) tract; monitoring fluid intake and output helps ensure adequate hydration and caloric intake.

10 Correct answer—B

Finger clubbing—thickening and flattening of the distal phalanges—results from the increased number of capillaries needed to enhance blood supply when chronic tissue hypoxia exists. Clubbing is common with disorders associated with chronic tissue hypoxia, such as congenital heart disease and cystic fibrosis. Acidosis, edema, and polycythemia do not cause finger clubbing. Children with congenital heart disease may have acidosis from insufficient tissue perfusion. Edema is a sign of congestive heart failure (CHF). Polycythemia may increase cardiac demands by increasing blood viscosity; this in turn may lead to CHF.

11 Correct answer—C

The nurse need not instruct parents to limit the child's activity level because children with TOF limit their own physical activity in response to decreased exercise tolerance. The body attempts to compensate for chronic hypoxia associated with cyanotic cardiac defects by increasing red blood cell (RBC) production, resulting in an elevated hematocrit and increasing blood viscosity. The knee-to-chest position may alleviate symptoms of hypoxic spells, thereby eliminating the incidence of recurrent spells. Dehydration exacerbates the increased blood viscosity and may be life-threatening. Children with TOF tire easily during feedings; therefore, small, frequent feedings are better tolerated.

12 Correct answer—A

Infants and children scheduled for cardiac catheterization must receive I.V. fluids to prevent dehydration and hypoglycemia. Oral fluids are withheld before surgery to reduce the risk of vomiting and aspiration. Electrocardiography, not electroencephalography, is performed before the procedure to monitor for arrhythmias. General anesthesia is avoided because of associated cardiovascular side effects. Oxygen administration is not a routine part of cardiac catheterization.

13 Correct answer—B

Restraining the arms and legs is the most common cause of injuries sustained during a seizure. Moving the child to the floor and removing sharp objects and furniture from the area can help prevent injuries. If the child has aspirated vomitus, medical help is needed as soon as possible to prevent hypoxia and aspiration pneumonia. The child should be turned onto the side to prevent the possibility of aspiration, and nothing should be forced into the mouth because this could damage the teeth. The time that the seizure began and ended and information about events preceding and following the seizure are especially important; such observations may help to identify precipitating factors that led to the seizure.

14 Correct answer—**A**

Mannitol (Osmitrol), an osmotic diuretic, is used to reduce increased intracranial pressure (ICP). Like other osmotic diuretics, mannitol increases intravascular osmolality, causing excess fluid in edematous tissues to move into the bloodstream. This action, in turn, reduces cerebral edema. Osmotic diuretics act rapidly and their effects last about 6 hours. Diphenhydramine (Benadryl) may be used to sedate a child with increased ICP. The diuretics hydrochlorothiazide (Aprozide) and furosemide (Lasix) are not used to treat increased ICP.

15 Correct answer—**B**

The nurse should avoid compressing the child's neck veins because this interferes with venous return and may exacerbate increased ICP. The bed should be elevated 15 to 30 degrees, with the child's head in a midline position to promote venous return. Mild range-of-motion exercises are indicated, and external stimuli should be minimized to help reduce ICP. Chest percussion and suctioning should be avoided because they increase ICP.

16 Correct answer—**B**

A word game, such as Scrabble, encourages a child to use cognitive skills, such as spelling and vocabulary. Kickball helps a child develop gross motor skills. Painting promotes fine motor skills. Building a tree fort promotes creativity and develops fine and gross motor skills.

17 Correct answer—**A**

Infants prefer to look at human faces rather than inanimate objects and focus best on objects 8″ to 10″ (20 to 25 cm) away. Although mobiles and objects with faces provide appropriate visual stimuli, those described here are not within the infant's focal range. An infant cannot focus on a television screen placed at the caregiver's viewing distance.

18 Correct answer—B

According to Erikson's theory, a school-age child who fails to master skills can develop feelings of inferiority. Displaying a child's art work around the unit without his permission may foster such feelings, especially if he does not feel his work is worthy of display. Praising the child for appropriate activities and encouraging group play or individual accomplishment through bedside play activities promote mastery of skills.

19 Correct answer—A

For a homozygous trait to occur, both parents, who are unaffected and heterozygous for that trait, must pass the defective gene or set of genes to the child. In each pregnancy, the child has a 25% chance of acquiring the trait, a 50% chance of being a carrier of the trait, and a 25% chance of being unaffected.

20 Correct answer—D

The most common complication of necrotizing enterocolitis (NEC) is intestinal perforation, which results from air in the intestinal lining produced by invading gas-forming organisms. Hydrocephalus, pneumothorax, and cholecystitis are unrelated to NEC.

21 Correct answer—D

The stools of an exclusively breast-fed neonate are yellowish and loose or watery and occur at nearly every feeding. Usually, they are nonirritating to the skin and pass easily. Because breast milk has a laxative effect during the first weeks after birth, stools may appear seedy or have the consistency of cottage cheese. In some cases, peristalsis slows and the neonate does not defecate for several days to a week; however, stool color and consistency should remain the same.

22 Correct answer—A

A neonate demonstrates the tonic neck reflex by extending the leg on the side to which the head is turned and flexing the contralateral (opposite) arm and leg (asymmetrical positioning). This reflex typically disappears by age 3 or 4 months, when symmetrical positioning (movement of the limbs in unison) occurs.

23 Correct answer—B

Screening for scoliosis, or lateral curvature of the spine, should be part of the physical examination of school-age children and adolescents. Scoliosis is a common problem in children, especially girls. Hip dysplasia (congenital hip dislocation) and osteogenesis imperfecta (a genetic disorder characterized by brittle, easily fractured bones) are congenital musculoskeletal abnormalities that appear at birth; both disorders are treated during infancy.

24 Correct answer—B

To help the child relax during an abdominal examination, the nurse should position the child with hips flexed and knees bent. Other appropriate measures include warming the hands before touching the child; palpating over the least tender areas first, using a gentle, circular motion and increasing palpation depth gradually; keeping the child covered during the examination; and telling the child what to expect by explaining or demonstrating on a doll beforehand.

25 Correct answer—D

Primary amenorrhea is delay of menarche after age 17. It results from abnormalities in the reproductive tract or endocrine system. Secondary amenorrhea refers to absence of menstruation for 12 months or more during the first 2 years after menarche or more than three consecutively missed periods thereafter. During the first 2 years after menarche, adolescents commonly miss one or two menstrual cycles; in many cases, this results from emotional disturbances.

26 Correct answer—C

Children rarely lie about sexual abuse; in fact, they typically have great difficulty talking about such sexual activities or abuse. Whether a child has a vivid imagination, masturbates, or feels jealous should not affect assessment.

27 Correct answer—D

Typically, weight gain associated with oral contraceptive use occurs cyclically from water retention; therefore, caloric intake should not be reduced. The dosage schedule, the medication's side effects, and the need for regular medical checkups should be included in a patient-teaching plan about oral contraceptives. This information allows the patient to take the medication safely while being aware of safeguards and potential side effects.

28 Correct answer—B

The peer group is crucial to development of an adolescent's self-image. Therefore, an adolescent prenatal group will provide peers to whom the teenager can relate and an opportunity to be accepted by a group. Group counseling can be effective even if participants are not in the same trimester of pregnancy. Individual counseling may leave the teenager feeling isolated and believing she is the only one going through this experience.

29 Correct answer—B

Because a child with cleft palate has structural deviations and alterations in muscle control, the eustachian tube may function inefficiently and permit drainage into the middle ear. This can cause increased pressure in the middle ear, recurrent otitis media, and tympanic membrane scarring. Therefore, hearing tests should be scheduled early and repeated throughout childhood, particularly when the child has a cold. Acoustic nerve immaturity, poor bone conduction, and congenital ear anomalies rarely are associated with cleft palate.

30 Correct answer—C

The infant should be placed in a prone position immediately after surgery to promote drainage of mucus and blood. This position also promotes drainage of oral secretions, helping to avoid the need for suction. The infant should remain in a prone position until the risk of secretion aspiration has decreased.

31 Correct answer—B

Speaking games, such as "pat-a-cake," and activities that encourage a child to imitate sounds promote normal speech development. Protecting the palate from speech movements is unnecessary. Drawing attention to the child's speech errors and correcting his speech may frustrate him. Reading stories enhances receptive language skills but does not reinforce expressive language (speech). Because much speech development is based on imitation, the parents should use appropriate speech forms, not baby talk, for the child to emulate.

32 Correct answer—**D**

Bleeding is a sign of esophagitis, which may manifest as hematemesis or occult blood in the stool or vomitus. A rattling cough in a child with gastroesophageal reflux (GER) results from repeated inhalation of gastric fluids, not esophagitis. Apnea, another complication of GER, is not associated with esophagitis. A child with GER may have apneic episodes with or without vomiting. Pallor would occur if the child became anemic.

33 Correct answer—**B**

A neonate in respiratory distress typically experiences tachycardia, not bradycardia, before becoming hypoxemic. Because the neonate breathes through the nose for the first 4 weeks after birth, nasal flaring signals respiratory distress. If lung compliance decreases and greater intrathoracic pressure is generated during inspiration, the neonate's chest wall may retract during inspiration.

34 Correct answer—**C**

Patients with anorexia nervosa have distorted and ambivalent perceptions of their bodies and commonly voice dislike of their physiques. They develop compulsive and ritualistic behaviors related to food to control their anxieties and hide their small food intake. This behavior may manifest as an intense interest in preparing and serving food. Their hunger awareness is inaccurate and they may claim to have no appetite. Typically, they increase their activity levels to counteract any possible weight gain and they exercise compulsively. Bingeing, fasting, and purging are associated with frequent weight fluctuations, which are characteristic in bulimia.

35 Correct answer—**D**

Anorexia nervosa involves a disturbance of body image and self-esteem, anxiety about meeting others' expectations, and a need to exert control. Because these underlying issues are related to family dynamics, therapy directed at these issues is appropriate. The other options can be implemented after therapy begins.

36 Correct answer—**A**

Decorticate posturing, a sign of cerebral cortex dysfunction, is characterized by adduction of the arms at the shoulders. The arms and wrists are flexed and form fists on the chest; the legs are adducted and extended.

37 Correct answer—D

Hyperbilirubinemia in a full-term neonate typically results from immature liver function and free hemoglobin that forms during RBC breakdown. This condition may lead to physiological jaundice, a form of jaundice arising 24 hours or more after birth and usually disappearing by the end of day 7. Yellow discoloration of the skin, sclerae, and gums is the chief sign. Polycythemia (an excessive number of RBCs), biliary atresia (obstruction or absence of the bile duct), and deficiency of the enzyme glucuronyl may contribute to hyperbilirubinemia; however, these are not the primary causes. In the liver, glucuronyl transferase helps conjugate bilirubin with glucuronic acid, making it more soluble.

38 Correct answer—A

Frequent and continual swallowing is the most obvious and early sign of postoperative hemorrhage—an occasional complication of tonsillectomy or adenoidectomy. Because blood oozing from the surgical site may be swallowed, a child may bleed heavily despite little apparent blood. Other signs of bleeding include frequent throat clearing, a pulse rate above 120 beats/minute, increased respirations, pallor, and restlessness. Hemorrhage may occur 5 to 10 days after surgery from tissue sloughing. The child may refuse to eat because of discomfort on swallowing; analgesics should be provided as needed. Headache is not a common postoperative complaint in this situation. Respiratory stridor—a harsh, high-pitched sound resulting from airway obstruction—also is not a typical postoperative complication.

39 Correct answer—B

Apple juice is a nonirritating clear liquid that will not be mistaken for blood—a possibility with pink and red beverages, such as grape or cherry soda. Milk and milk products should not be given because they are viscous and will cause frequent throat clearing, which may trigger bleeding at the surgical site. Fruit juices, especially citrus juices, should be avoided because they may irritate the throat. The child can begin a soft diet on the first or second postoperative day. Eating increases blood supply to the tissues, promoting healing.

40 Correct answer—A

A barium enema usually has no role in evaluating Hodgkin's disease. The erythrocyte sedimentation rate (ESR), gallium scan, and chest X-ray are part of the usual workup. An elevated ESR is common in cancer patients. A gallium scan can be used to determine whether cancer has metastasized to the bone; a chest X-ray can help determine whether it has spread to the lungs.

41 Correct answer—D

Protocols for care of a central venous line vary with the health care facility. However, a reduced-strength heparin solution of 10 units/ml or 100 units/ml typically is used as a final flush to prevent clotting and maintain catheter patency. Full-strength heparin solutions are not used because they can cause systemic heparinization. A normal saline flush is insufficient to prevent the catheter from clotting.

42 Correct answer—D

Hyperbilirubinemia in a full-term neonate typically results from immature liver function and free hemoglobin that forms during RBC breakdown. This condition may lead to physiologic jaundice, a form of jaundice arising 24 hours or more after birth and usually disappearing by the end of day 7. Yellow discoloration of the skin, sclerae, and gums is the chief sign. Polycythemia (an excessive number of RBCs), biliary atresia (obstruction or absence of the bile duct), and deficiency of the enzyme glucuronyl may contribute to hyperbilirubinemia; however, these are not the primary causes. In the liver, glucuronyl transferase helps conjugate bilirubin with glucoronic acid, making it more soluble.

43 Correct answer—A

Calcium levels are highest in broccoli, kale, and mustard and turnip greens, as well as in dairy products, sardines, and salmon bones. Calcium is essential for bone growth and development, blood clotting, and neuromuscular function. Children need about 800 mg of calcium daily.

44 Correct answer—C

The initial step in health education involves assessing an individual's needs, motivation, developmental level, knowledge base, and learning ability. By asking such open-ended questions as, "What do you know about toilet training?" the nurse can elicit information and provide a basis for more specific questions that can lead to teaching. Questions involving the caregiver's previous experience and motivation and the child's readiness for toilet training should be part of the assessment phase, but these questions are too specific to be of value initially.

45 Correct answer—B

Infant-caregiver interaction is best assessed during feeding. The way in which the caregiver holds the infant and looks at his face provides clues about her anxiety level and overall feelings for the child. Likewise, the infant's posture and responses to the caregiver provide clues about his comfort level and feelings. During feeding, the caregiver holds the infant within 12″ to 15″ of eye level. This distance seems most comfortable for the caregiver and provides the infant with optimal visual stimulation. Sleep periods do not provide an opportunity for infant-caregiver interaction. Although playing and rocking provide clues about developing infant-caregiver interaction, they are not the primary method of assessing such an exchange.

46 Correct answer—B

In pubescent boys, pubic hair begins to develop at the base of the penis and eventually grows over the entire pubic region. The inguinal area, which contains lymphatic glands, usually is not covered with pubic hair.

47 Correct answer—C

Before initiating chest compression in an infant, the nurse should visualize a line between the infant's nipples. She then should place two or three fingers on the sternum one finger-width below the imaginary line; this is the correct hand placement for performing cardiopulmonary resuscitation on a child under age 1. An infant's heart is positioned more horizontally than an adult's, and the apex is higher (at the third or fourth intercostal space versus the fifth intercostal space in an older child or adult). Placing the hands above or below the designated landmark results in less effective cardiac compressions. Hand placement at the xiphoid could result in fracture and subsequent internal injuries.

48 Correct answer—**A**

Appendicitis (inflammation of the appendix)—the most common cause of pediatric abdominal surgery—can occur in all age-groups, but it rarely occurs in children under age 2. Untreated appendicitis can result in peritonitis. Phimosis is a narrowing of the foreskin opening; surgical repair (indicated in only severe cases) involves circumcision, which is not considered abdominal surgery. Inguinal hernia repair is the most common surgical procedure in infants. Hydrocele—a circumscribed collection of fluid typically found in the testicle or along the spermatic cord—usually resolves spontaneously; surgery is not required unless the hydrocele persists beyond age 1.

49 Correct answer—**D**

Polyuria, polydipsia, weight loss, and nocturia or nocturnal enuresis are caused by a lack of adequate insulin secretion. These symptoms commonly occur at the onset of diabetes in children. Polyuria, nocturia, or nocturnal enuresis are caused by hyperglycemia, which leads to osmotic diuresis. This diuresis causes dehydration, which leads to polydipsia. Weight loss occurs when body tissues break down to meet energy requirements. The presence of glucose in the urine is responsible for a high specific gravity.

50 Correct answer—**C**

When assessing a child with a suspected respiratory tract infection, the nurse must note any contributing factors, including the child's nutritional status, living conditions and sanitation, exposure to illness or disease, delays in immunizations, travel, and results of tuberculin tests. These factors provide data about the possible causes of the infection. Subsequent interventions and treatment, such as respiratory isolation and antibiotic therapy, are based on the cause of the infection. The nurse also must assess the child's hydration status because dehydration is associated with respiratory tract infections; however, this information is not as important as identifying the cause of infection. An assessment of surrounding vegetation is pertinent when allergic rhinitis or asthma is suspected. School activity is irrelevant in this situation.

51 Correct answer—**B**

For lumbar puncture, an infant should be placed in an arched position to maximize the space between the L3 and L5 vertebrae. The nurse's hands should rest on the back of the infant's shoulders to prevent neck flexion, which could block the airway and cause respiratory arrest. The infant should be at the edge of the bed or table during the procedure, and the nurse should speak quietly to calm him. A mummy restraint limits access to the lumbar area because it involves snugly wrapping the child's trunk and extremities in a blanket or towel; this restraint is appropriate for procedures involving the head or neck because it leaves only these body parts exposed. A prone position would not separate the vertebral spaces.

52 Correct answer—**D**

A hemangioma is a red birthmark with a rough surface that may be present at birth or appear during the first month after delivery. It disappears spontaneously in childhood and is not related to cerebral palsy. During physical assessment of an infant with suspected cerebral palsy, the nurse should stay alert for sensory deficits (such as vision, hearing, and speech problems), persistence of primitive reflexes (particularly an asymmetrical tonic neck reflex and a crossed extension reflex), and signs of impaired arm or leg movement. The nurse also should evaluate the infant's feeding skills, motor development, muscle tone, range of motion, weight, vital signs, and level of consciousness. Motor dysfunction may not become apparent until the infant acquires more advanced skills, such as standing.

53 Correct answer—**C**

Cerebral palsy, a nonspecific term for impaired muscle function, is classified according to the nature of the disorder. The spastic quadriplegia form of cerebral palsy—the most common form—is characterized by tense, contracted muscles. Athetoid (dyskinetic) cerebral palsy is characterized by constant uncontrolled movements. Mixed cerebral palsy, a combination of the spastic and athetoid forms, is characterized by spasticity, facial grimacing, writhing, and flailing. A poor sense of balance and depth perception is associated with ataxic cerebral palsy. Rigid, tremor, and atonic types of cerebral palsy are uncommon.

54 Correct answer—C

Only the question "Does she hop and run?" elicits information specific to the child's gross motor development. The other questions involve sensory or cognitive development.

55 Correct answer—A

Refusing to place the child in an appropriate special education program should alert the nurse to the possibility that the mother has not accepted her daughter's diagnosis. However, before drawing any conclusions, the nurse should determine whether the mother is unhappy with the particular program. Then the nurse should evaluate the need for further intervention. Viewing the child as whole rather than focusing on the defect, recognizing the child's fatigue level during therapy, and participating in a parental support group would demonstrate acceptance of the diagnosis.

56 Correct answer—B

A nursing diagnosis of *Feeding self-care deficit related to neuromuscular impairment* would be supported by the child's inability to bring food from plate to mouth. Although inaccurate interpretation of environmental stimuli and swallowing only liquid foods may be related to neuromuscular impairment, they do not reflect the child's ability to feed herself. Dislike of many foods is unrelated to neuromuscular impairment or self-feeding.

57 Correct answer—A

The nurse can foster the child's positive self-image most effectively by discussing with family members the importance of accepting her. Support and acceptance from significant others can motivate a disabled child to work hard and develop skills. Encouraging the child's social interaction with peers also is necessary but is not the best intervention in this situation. Family is the most influential force for a 5-year-old child; peer acceptance rarely is a major factor until the child reaches school age. Noting signs of grieving or depression is important; however, it only alerts the nurse to the child's negative feelings and does not provide an immediate solution. Encouraging the child to avoid discussing her disability is inappropriate; avoidance or denial will not make the problem go away.

58 Correct answer—C

Lonnie is susceptible to infection because of a low white blood cell (WBC) count—specifically a low absolute neutrophil count. Neutrophils are phagocytes that ingest foreign substances and play a key role in preventing infections. Lonnie is neither anemic (hemoglobin value below 10 g/dl) by oncology transfusion standards nor thrombocytopenic (platelet count above 100,000 mm^3. She also is not particularly susceptible to stroke; her risk of stroke would be increased if she had an extremely high WBC count because in this situation, WBCs sludge, causing ischemia or infarction.

59 Correct answer—A

Lonnie should avoid crowds only when her absolute neutrophil count falls below 500 mm^3. If her platelet count is below 50,000 mm^3, she is susceptible to injury and bleeding and should avoid contact sports or activities that can cause injury or bleeding, such as bicycle riding, skateboarding, and gymnastics. A low neutrophil count would necessitate minimizing the risk for infection, not avoiding school, sports, or physicial activities. Hand washing is an important aspect of infection control; however, a protective mask is not necessary during neutropenic episodes. Children with cancer should not receive immunizations for at least 3 months after chemotherapy; this delay allows the immune system to recover sufficiently and respond appropriately to the vaccine. Live vaccines, such as polio and measles-mumps-rubella vaccines, must be avoided because they can cause overwhelming infection in a child with a depressed immune system.

60 Correct answer—D

False reassurance is inappropriate, especially for a child with cancer. Aspects of cancer treatment that can frighten a 5-year-old child include bone marrow aspiration, lumbar puncture, and frequent venipuncture. Hospitalization also can be a frightening experience. Intense nausea, vomiting, and hair loss are anxiety-producing side effects of chemotherapy. The most important intervention is to explain the disease and its treatment to Lonnie in terms she can understand. Playing with a toy medical kit may help her release some of her anxieties and resentment. The nurse should allow Lonnie to choose which leg will receive the injection so that she will feel she has some control over her situation.

61 Correct answer—C

Most children with leukemia receive treatment for 2½ to 3 years (although this may vary). The extended treatment period is needed to achieve a prolonged remission or cure because leukemic cells that were not destroyed may hide in the bone marrow or other parts of the body, multiplying quickly and causing a relapse. The consolidation phase that follows induction involves different chemotherapeutic agents to kill the cancerous cells that survived initial treatment. Therapy also is designed specifically to target cells that may be hiding in body tissues, such as the CNS. These cells may not be detected by blood tests, bone marrow aspiration, and cerebrospinal fluid examination. Prognosis is determined by the type of leukemia and other data, such as the patient's age, initial WBC count, and cell morphology. Lonnie's diagnosis and age favor a positive prognosis. Such responses as, "That's the way her protocol is designed" and "Research shows that..." provide little explanation about why the treatment should be continued.

62 Correct answer—D

Early identification of an eating disorder, which can be devastating and extremely hard to treat, promotes a positive outcome. Clinicians recommend assessing all preadolescent and adolescent girls with suspected eating disorders in the following areas: problems in personality structure and related behaviors, such as signs of low self-esteem, high achievement without a sense of competence, and external loss of control; problems with body image, such as a belief that specific body parts are obese or distorted in some way; problems with weight and food-related behaviors, such as food rituals, the belief that some foods are "good" and others "bad," compulsive exercising, and frequent weighings; and problems with family dynamics, such a history of eating disorders, substance abuse, affective disorders, intrusive control, or marital discord. Assessing an adolescent's athletic achievements may be helpful but is not a major way to identify an eating disorder.

63 Correct answer—B

Fluid and electrolyte imbalances are serious complications of eating disorders. Electrolyte screening may reveal metabolic alkalosis, increased sodium and chloride levels, and potassium deficiency. Unlike the anorectic patient, whose condition only deteriorates, the bulimic adolescent maintains a delicate fluid and electrolyte balance and suddenly may develop impending or frank shock, severe hypokalemia, cardiac arrhythmias, acute renal failure, seizures, or acute gastric dilatation or rupture. Diarrhea or anemia may result from purging or malnourishment; however, these conditions are not as dangerous as electrolyte abnormalities. Diabetes is not a complication of bulimia.

64 Correct answer—A

A common personality trait among bulimic patients is low self-esteem. Bulimic behavior typically begins in adolescence, when self-esteem is most threatened. Bulimic patients feel out of control and experience internal mood states of anger, boredom, depression, anxiety, and hunger. Their perceived lack of control causes greater dissatisfaction and they become enraged at their bodies, which they view as imperfect or defective. Because bulimic patients have high expectations of themselves, they suffer from persistent guilt, shame, and self-criticism. Aggression, assertiveness, and creativity are not characteristic of patients with bulimia.

65 Correct answer—C

Cystic fibrosis is a genetic disorder of the exocrine (mucus-producing) glands. A family history of cystic fibrosis would alert the nurse to a possible diagnosis of this disease. Other suggestive findings include increased sweat electrolyte levels, absence of pancreatic enzymes, and chronic pulmonary involvement. Children with cystic fibrosis typically excrete large amounts of fat in the stool (steatorrhea) from impaired fat absorption.

66 Correct answer—C

Because cystic fibrosis impairs GI absorption, dietary planning focuses on providing adequate caloric intake. Dietary fat content may need to be restricted if steatorrhea is not controlled by enzyme replacement; however, a fat-free diet is not necessary. Absence of pancreatic enzymes compromises fat and protein digestion and absorption. Therefore, pancreatic enzyme replacement (Pancrease or Cotazym-S) is indicated. Impaired fat absorption hinders absorption of the fat-soluble vitamins A, D, E, and K; consequently, taking a water-miscible daily multivitamin would be appropriate. In some cases, medium-chain triglycerides are given as a supplement because they are absorbed more readily than long-chain fats. During hot weather, febrile illness, or strenuous exercise, sodium is depleted through sweating. Therefore, children with cystic fibrosis should use salt liberally.

67 Correct answer—C

Phenylketonuria (PKU) is a genetic disorder characterized by inability to metabolize phenylalanine, an amino acid found in foods containing protein. Normally, phenylalanine is converted to tyrosine by the enzyme phenylalanine hydroxylase. This enzyme is absent in children with PKU, leading to phenylalanine accumulation. Dietary protein is the body's phenylalanine source; if the diet is not altered, CNS irritability and mental retardation may occur. Because phenylalanine is an essential amino acid required for growth, it cannot be completely eliminated from the diet; the child must ingest small amounts to maintain therapeutic blood levels. However, high-protein foods, such as meats and dairy products, are restricted or eliminated from the diet. Infants with PKU commonly receive the formula Lofenalac.

68 Correct answer—D

A large, soft anterior fontanel and large tongue appear in infants with congenital hypothyroidism, not PKU. Neonates with PKU exhibit irritability, vomiting, hyperactivity, and unpredictable behavior. These signs relate to phenylalanine accumulation, which adversely affects development of the CNS. Defective myelinization and degeneration of white and gray matter also occur. Infants with PKU typically have fair skin (from absence of tyramine, which is needed for pigment formation) and are prone to dermatologic problems, especially eczema. Phenylalanine accumulation causes urinary excretion of phenyl acids, abnormal metabolites that give the urine a musty odor.

69 Correct answer—B

Signs and symptoms of aminophylline toxicity include an increased heart rate, restlessness, insomnia, nervousness, twitching, seizures, and hyperactive reflexes. Aminophylline prevents breakdown of adenylcyclase, an adrenergic activator; consequently, manifestations of aminophylline toxicity reflect increased adrenergic activity.

70 Correct answer—B

Asthma is a controllable disease. Appropriate medications, environmental control, teaching, and crisis planning can help the patient participate in normal daily activities and achieve personal goals. It is not always possible to wean an asthmatic child from medication or to prevent upper respiratory tract infections or asthma attacks.

71 Correct answer—C

Remaining calm will allow the patient with asthma to think clearly and contribute to more effective respiratory effort. Various relaxation techniques, including controlled breathing, can help during the attack. Drinking tepid fluids maintains hydration and prevents bronchial mucus from becoming too viscous. Cold fluids should be avoided because they may precipitate bronchospasm. Albuterol administered via inhalation starts to exert its bronchodilatory effect within 15 minutes. If these self-management procedures do not provide relief within a reasonable time (usually within 20 minutes), Grace should be taken to the emergency department.

72 Correct answer—D

Tracheoesophageal fistula (TEF) is a rare but serious malformation representing failure of the esophagus to develop as a continuous passage to the stomach. The esophagus may consist of two blind pouches—one at the pharyngeal end and one at the gastric end. More often, however, one portion ends in a blind pouch and the other is connected to the trachea by way of a fistula. Esophageal atresia with a blind upper pouch and a fistula from the lower pouch to the trachea is the most common form of this anomaly. A neonate with TEF typically exhibits choking, sneezing, and coughing of excessive mucus. Cyanosis may occur at feedings. Respiratory secretions typically are increased; breaths may be diminished if the child develps pneumonia. Abdominal distention and visible peristalsis would not be noted because of the absence of a continuous passage to the stomach and GI tract. Projectile vomiting and increased bowel sounds are indicative of a bowel obstruction; they are unrelated to TEF.

73 Correct answer—C

The neonate should not be fed orally until the physician makes a definitive diagnosis. Oral feedings markedly increase the risk of aspiration because this neonate lacks a direct route to the stomach and has abnormal communication between the esophagus and trachea. Nasogastric feedings are inappropriate because the neonate's esophagus ends in a blind pouch or connects to the trachea via a fistula. The neonate should be given I.V. fluids and kept in an upright position to prevent the reflux of gastric juices from the fistula into the lungs.

74 Correct answer—B

Keeping the neonate supine with the head of the crib elevated at least 30 degrees helps prevent aspiration and regurgitation of gastric contents through the fistula into the trachea.

75 Correct answer—C

Because the likelihood of aspiration is high in a neonate with TEF, the nurse should keep suction equipment—suction machine, suction catheter, sterile gloves, and sterile saline solution—readily available. A bulb syringe is insufficient for the depth and amount of suctioning required for this neonate. Although the airway should be cleared of secretions, an artificial airway and tracheostomy set are not needed for this purpose.

76 Correct answer—C

Chemical pneumonitis, or pneumonia, is an inflammation of the lung caused by irritating substances, such as those present in gastric contents. Aspiration of bronchial and gastric secretions is a constant concern of nurses who care for infants with TEF. The severity of chemical pneumonitis determines the treatment approach. NEC is characterized by a severely decreased blood supply to the intestine that causes ischemia. An ischemic bowel associated with excessive formula in the intestinal lumen and bacterial colonization signal development of NEC. Bronchopulmonary dysplasia is a chronic lung disorder that develops in neonates with lung disease who are exposed to high oxygen concentrations and positive pressure ventilation. An anorectal anomaly may occur in any neonate and is not related to TEF.

77 Correct answer—B

The two tests used to detect antibodies to human immunodeficiency virus (HIV)—the virus that causes acquired immunodeficiency (AIDS)—are the enzyme-linked immunosorbent assay (ELISA) and the Western blot. Both tests provide fast, accurate results. The Wasserman test is used to diagnose syphilis. AZT (zidovudine) is a medication used to treat patients with AIDS.

78 Correct answer—A

The Centers for Disease Control's diagnostic criteria for children with AIDS are the presence of certain risk factors (such as a mother who is an I.V. drug abuser or contact with blood or body fluids of an infected person), the presence of an opportunistic infection, and the absence of other immunodeficiency diseases.

79 Correct answer—A

A detailed history outlining frequent infections and a thorough physical assessment are necessary follow-up measures for a child who is diagnosed with AIDS. Physical assessment provides baseline data against which future changes can be evaluated; it may reveal such abnormalities as neuropathy, cardiopathy, and hepatosplenitis. Although some genetic pools and social or cultural groups are predisposed to certain diseases (for example, African Americans are predisposed to cardiovascular disease, Mexican Americans to pneumonia), no such association exists with AIDS. All people infected with HIV are at high risk for AIDS.

80 Correct answer—A

Children with AIDS typically develop slowly and may regress developmentally. Whether this results from the AIDS virus or psychosocial factors is unknown. A diagnostic workup for a child with AIDS should include a comprehensive baseline developmental assessment, which should be repeated every 6 months to 1 year to determine if developmental skills have deteriorated. Because AIDS affects a child's physical and psychosocial development, this assessment typically addresses physical, psychological, and social development. Various pediatric developmental assessment tools are available, such as the Denver Developmental Screening Tests and Questionnaires, the Developmental Profile, and the McCarthy Developmental Scales of Children's Abilities.

81 Correct answer—D

Misinformation or lack of knowledge is the main reason why some health care workers refuse to care for AIDS patients. Therefore, the nurse-manager should educate and counsel Sandra about this disease. Allowing her to refuse to care for Maria would set a precedent for all nurses who do not want to care for AIDS patients. The Code for Nurses does not allow discrimination against a patient based on illness. A nurse can refuse to participate in care only on the grounds of patient advocacy or moral objection to a specific intervention. Assigning Sandra to another unit does not address the problem and only serves to reinforce her misinformation.

82 Correct answer—C

Calorie counting is an effective tool for determining dietary intake on both a daily and an extended basis. Average daily caloric requirements for children are as follows:

Age	Calories/kg of weight
Both sexes	
0-6 months	115
6-12 months	105
1-3 year	100
4-6 years	85
7-10 years	85
Boys	
11-14 years	60
15-18 years	42
Girls	
11-14 years	48
15-18 years	38

Caloric requirements for children with AIDS have not been defined quantitatively. However, fever, stress from opportunistic infections, diarrhea, and vomiting increase the need for calories. The child's birth weight has no bearing on current dietary intake. Daily weight and fluid intake and output measurements help assess hydration status.

83 Correct answer—D

The physician performs bronchoscopy to determine the type of pneumonia. In bronchoscopy, a flexible tube (bronchoscope) is passed through the mouth or nose to the lower respiratory tract to visualize the tracheobronchial tree. Culture specimens are obtained by threading a brush through the bronchoscope to the affected area and brushing the tissue to collect pathogens (brush biopsy). *Pneumocystis carinii* pneumonia and chronic candidiasis are the most common opportunistic infections associated with AIDS. Other opportunistic infections of the respiratory tract include *Cryptococcus,* histoplasmosis, and *Mycobacterium* tuberculosis. Nothing in the situation suggests the possibility of a mucus plug or the need for bronchial lavage. The extent of pneumonia would be determined by X-ray and physical assessment findings.

84 Correct answer—D

The nurse should observe universal (barrier) precautions, which include blood and body fluid precautions, when caring for all patients—especially those with diagnosed or suspected AIDS. These precautions are needed because HIV is transmitted via the blood and body fluids. Universal precautions include wearing gloves for direct contact with body substances; wearing a gown when spillage on clothing is anticipated; wearing a mask when diseases spread by the respiratory route are known or suspected; and wearing a mask and eye coverings when exposure to mucous membranes is foreseen. Because HIV may be present in any body fluid or secretion, isolation techniques (such as respiratory, enteric, or blood precautions) are insufficient to protect the nurse from all potential sources of exposure.

85 Correct answer—B

Impaired gas exchange related to respiratory infection is the major reason for Maria's hospitalization. Although children with AIDS commonly have diarrhea, nothing in the situation suggests that Maria has this problem. Children with failure to thrive may be at risk for *Impaired skin integrity related to poor nutritional status,* but no evidence indicates that Maria has this problem. Also, no evidence suggests that Maria has impaired mobility.

86 Correct answer—C

Maria is experiencing failure to thrive, a term used to describe the condition of a child whose weight (and sometimes height) is below the fifth percentile for her age. Children with AIDS may experience organic failure to thrive (related to a physiological disturbance, such as chronic diarrhea) or nonorganic failure to thrive (related to adverse psychosocial factors, such as disturbance in the maternal-infant relationship stemming from the mother's drug abuse). Total parenteral nutrition (TPN; also called hyperalimentation) refers to parenteral administration of fluid, calories, and nutrients through a large vein. It provides total or supplemental calories for patients who cannot consume sufficient calories through the alimentary tract. TPN solutions are prescribed individually according to the patient's nutritional needs; typically, they contain glucose, protein, vitamins, and minerals. TPN will increase Maria's caloric intake and help her gain weight; it is not intended to increase her fluid intake. It also does not reduce the risk of infections; in fact, it may increase this risk because use of a central venous access device to administer the solution provides a portal of entry for microorganisms and serves as an excellent medium for bacterial growth. Parenteral medications are not mixed with TPN solutions; they should be administered via separate I.V. access.

87 Correct answer—A

Including play as part of a child's daily routine is an important component of pediatric nursing care. Play provides a child with an outlet for fear and other emotions. Blocks are an appropriate toy for Maria because they allow her to vent her frustrations and are easy to clean. They also can help her develop motor skills and visual coordination—necessary developmental milestones for a 2-year-old. A child of Maria's age lacks the fine motor skills needed to string beads, and the beads may pose a choking hazard. Because a 2-year-old typically has little control over respiratory secretions and tends to put objects in the mouth, toys that are hard to clean (such as puzzles and stuffed animals) are inappropriate.

88 Correct answer—B

Diarrhea, caused by reduction in intestinal bacteria, is a common side effect of antibiotic therapy. The nurse should report diarrhea to the physician; in some cases, therapy will be discontinued or modified. Decreased appetite, stomach pain, and vomiting also are associated with antibiotic therapy but occur less frequently than diarrhea.

89 Correct answer—D

When preparing Maria for discharge, the nurse should observe the primary caregiver to assess the caregiver's ability to meet the child's physical and emotional needs and to reinforce the child's needs with her family. The physician and pharmacist arrange for outpatient medication; the nurse's role is to teach family members about medication administration and side effects. Arranging for transportation home usually is the social worker's responsibility. Hospices play a role in caring for AIDS patients in the terminal disease stage; because Maria has not reached this stage, a referral at this time would be inappropriate. However, the nurse should assist the social worker in arranging for services Maria and her family may need after discharge, including visiting nurse services, outpatient therapy, and support groups. AIDS should be viewed as a chronic disorder that requires extensive follow-up care.

90 Correct answer—D

Education is the key to allaying fears and misconceptions about AIDS. To devise an effective teaching plan, the nurse should evaluate the family's knowledge of the disease. The nurse can reduce family members' anxiety by explaining how AIDS is transmitted and discussing specific measures to prevent transmission. The family may need instructions on basic infection control measures, such as thorough hand washing and proper handling of secretions and contaminated articles. The nurse should assure family members that they can share the same kitchen, bathroom, and sleeping facilities with the patient because no cases of AIDS from casual contact have been reported. The nurse can act as role model by touching the patient when providing care. Planning a home assessment visit, arranging a meeting with the family of another AIDS patient, and encouraging participation in support groups will not address the family's fears and concerns.

91 Correct answer—D

Maria's compromised immune system places her at increased risk for contracting respiratory or gastric infections from others. The only measure that specifically decreases the risk of infection is keeping her away from people with infections. Although the physician may prescribe vitamin and mineral supplements to promote nutrition and correct any dietary deficiencies, these substances are not a major means of preventing infection. Scheduling regular clinic visits and providing a balanced diet may contribute to the child's optimal health.

92 Correct answer—C

A child with AIDS should be evaluated whenever an infection is suspected because any infection may be life-threatening. A child with AIDS tends to develop serious infections from poor antibody production and destruction of B lymphocytes (which produce antibodies) by HIV. Overwhelming bacterial infections account for much of the mortality among pediatric AIDS patients. Therefore, the caregiver should seek medical attention as soon as an infection is suspected. The other options might be appropriate for a child who does not have AIDS; however, because of Maria's immunocompromised status, further evaluation is warranted.

93 Correct answer—B

Maria should be encouraged to lead the most normal life-style possible to promote growth and development. Although her grandmother's need to overprotect her is understandable, the nurse should encourage her to express her fears and concerns so that they may be addressed. Maria need not be restricted from playing with other children.

94 Correct answer—B

Bulging fontanels indicate increased intracranial pressure and is the most significant finding in infants and young children with meningitis. This sign commonly is accompanied by a high-pitched cry. An infant with meningitis may display nuchal rigidity. Kernig's sign and photophobia are hard to assess in extremely young children, who may be uncooperative or too frightened to permit a thorough examination. Heart sounds are unrelated to meningitis.

95 Correct answer—A

A child with meningitis is isolated for the first 24 hours or until culture results identify the causative organism. Respiratory isolation, which requires the use of a mask, gown, and good handwashing technique, usually is necessary for 24 hours after antimicrobial therapy begins. Precautions are needed to protect the nurse and others from possible infection. Protective isolation (described in option C) or reverse isolation (described in option D) is not indicated in these cases. Wearing gloves when changing diapers adheres to enteric precautions, which are unnecessary in this situation.

96 Correct answer—D

A child with meningitis has increased intracranial pressure; over-hydrating the child would further increase the pressure, resulting in cerebral edema. Therefore, careful monitoring of intake and output is necessary in a child with meningitis to prevent cerebral edema and other problems associated with fluid accumulation. Keeping an infant slightly dehydrated decreases the risk of cerebral edema. Circulatory overload, electrolyte imbalance, and kidney failure are not related to meningitis.

97 Correct answer—B

A positive test result for HIV indicates that the patient has been exposed to the human immunodeficiency virus and has developed antibodies against it. Diagnosis of AIDS-related complex is based on a positive result to HIV testing, the appearance of symptoms associated with AIDS with no apparant signs of an opportunistic infection, and classification as a member of a high-risk group. Currently, no definitive test is available to diagnose the presence of the AIDS virus.

98 Correct answer—D

Many misconceptions exist about AIDS. For example, many people fear they will contract AIDS through casual contact. Evaluating the parents' level of knowledge about the disease is crucial to devising an effective education plan. AIDS is not a common complication of hemophilia; it is a disease transmitted through contact with infected blood or body fluids. The nurse should stress to the parents that other family members are not at risk for acquiring the AIDS virus as long as they adhere to blood and body fluid precautions.

99 Correct answer—C

All health care workers should wear gloves when handling blood and body secretions to prevent HIV transmission. In this situation, the school nurse and Christopher's teacher should take whatever measures are necessary to control the bleeding—while wearing gloves. Allowing the bleeding to stop spontaneously would be inappropriate because of the child's increased risk for hemorrhage from the absence of clotting factors. Although notifying Christopher's parents and physician is important, the primary objective is to stop the bleeding.

100 Correct answer—**B**

A solution of 1 part of chlorine bleach to 10 parts of water will disinfect surfaces contaminated by HIV-infected body fluids.

Selected references

Chapter 1

Church, J.L., and Baer, K.J. "Examination of the Adolescent: A Practical Guide," *Journal of Pediatric Health Care* 1(2):65-72, March/April 1987.

Denholm, C., and Ferguson, R. "Strategies to Promote the Developmental Needs of Hospitalized Adolescents," *Children's Health Care* 15(3):183-87, Winter 1987.

Dickey, S.B. *A Guide to the Nursing of Children.* Baltimore: Williams & Wilkens Co., 1987.

Haylor, M. "Human Response to Loss," *Nurse Practitioner* 12(2):63-66, May 1987.

James, S., and Mott, S. *Child Health Nursing Essential Care of Children and Families.* Reading, Mass.: Addison-Wesley Publishing Co., 1988.

Lowery, G.H. *Growth and Development of Children,* 8th ed. Chicago: Year Book Medical Publishers, 1986.

Marlow, D., and Redding, B. *Textbook of Pediatric Nursing,* 6th ed. Philadelphia: W.B. Saunders Co., 1988.

McCue, K. "Medical Play: An Expanded Perspective," *Children's Health Care* 16(3):157-61, Winter 1988.

Mott, S.R., et al. *Nursing Care of Children and Families: A Holistic Approach,* 2nd ed. Menlo Park, Calif.: Addison-Wesley Publishing Co., 1990.

Muscari, M. "Obtaining the Adolescent Sexual History," *Pediatric Nursing* 13(5):307-10, September/October 1987.

Rhyme, M. "Understanding and Supporting Families in the Process of Divorce," *Nurse Practitioner* 11(12):37-51, December 1986.

Scharf, M. *Waking Up Dry: How to End Bedwetting Forever.* Cincinnati: Writer's Digest Books, 1986.

Schuster, C., and Ashburn, S. *The Process of Human Development,* 2nd ed. Glenview, Ill.: Scott-Forseman, 1986.

Scipien, G.M., et al. *Comprehensive Pediatric Nursing,* 3rd ed. New York: McGraw-Hill Book Co., 1986.

Whaley, L.F., and Wong, D.L. *Nursing Care of Infants and Children,* 4th ed. St. Louis: Mosby-Year Book, 1991.

Chapter 2

Avery, G. *Neonatology: Pathophysiology and Management of the Newborn,* 3rd ed. Philadelphia: J.B. Lippincott Co., 1987.

Gaffney, S.E., and Salinger, L. "Group B Streptococcus: The Pregnant Woman and Her Neonate," *JOGNN* 16(2):91-96, March/April 1987.

Klaus, M.H., and Fanaroff, A.A. *Care of the High-Risk Neonate,* 3rd ed. Philadelphia: W.B. Saunders Co., 1986.

Korones, S.B. *High-Risk Newborn Infants,* 4th ed. St. Louis: C.V. Mosby Co., 1986.

Streeter, N.S. *High-Risk Neonatal Care.* Rockville, Md.: Aspen Systems, 1986.

Weibley, T.T., et al. "Gavage Tube Insertion in the Premature Infant," *MCN* 12(1):24-27, January/February 1987.

Chapter 3

Dixon, S.D., and Stein, M.T. *Encounters with Children: Pediatric Behavior and Development.* Chicago: Year Book Medical Publishers, 1987.

Raish, P., and Klaus, B. *Every Nurse's Guide to Physical Assessment: A Primary Care Focus.* New York: John Wiley & Sons, 1987.

Servonsky, J., and Opas, S. *Nursing Management of Children.* Boston: Jones & Bartlett Publishers, 1987.

Whaley, L.F., and Wong, D.L. *Nursing Care of Infants and Children,* 3rd ed. St. Louis: C.V. Mosby Co., 1986.

Chapter 4

Alfaro, R. *Applying Nursing Diagnosis & Nursing Process,* 2nd ed. Philadelphia: J.B. Lippincott Co., 1990.

Bates, B. *A Guide to Physical Examination and History Taking,* 5th ed. Philadelphia: J.B. Lippincott Co., 1991.

Beischer, N.A., and Mackay, E.V. *Obstetrics and the Newborn.* Philadlephia: W.B. Saunders Co., 1986.

Fox, S.I. *Human Physiology,* 2nd ed. Dubuque, Iowa: William C. Brown, 1987.

Fullar, S.A. "Care of Postpartum Adolescents," *MCN* 11(6):398-403, November/December 1986.

Jensen, M., and Bobak, I. *Maternity and Gynecologic Care,* 4th ed. St. Loius: C.V. Mosby Co., 1989.

Johnson, S.H., ed. *Nursing Assessment and Strategies for the Family at Risk: High Risk Parenting,* 2nd ed. Philadelphia: J.B. Lippincott Co., 1986.

Konrad, C. "Helping Mothers Integrate the Birth Experience," *MCN* 12(4):268-69, July/August 1987.

Schwartz, M.W., et al. *Principles and Practice of Clinical Pediatrics.* Chicago: Year Book Medical Publishers, 1987.

Servonsky, J., and Opas, S. *Nursing Management of Children.* Boston: Jones & Barlett Publishing Co., 1987.

Stanhope, M., and Lancaster, J. *Community Health Nursing,* 2nd ed. St. Louis: C.V. Mosby Co., 1988.

Yoos, L. "Adolescent Cognitive and Contraceptive Behaviors," *Pediatric Nursing* 13(4):247-50, July/August 1987.

Chapter 5

Keller, O.L. "Bulimia: Primary Care Approach and Intervention," *Nurse Practitioner* 11(8):42-51, August 1986.

Muscari, M.E. "Identification and Management of the Early Anorectic Child," *Journal of Pediatric Health Care* 1(4):196-203, July/August 1987.

Neinstein, L. *Adolescent Health Care,* 2nd ed. Baltimore: Urban & Schwartzenberg, 1990.

Chapter 6

American Academy of Pediatrics Committee on Infectious Diseases. "Health Guidelines for the Attendance in Day Care and Foster Care Settings of Children Infected with Human Immunodeficiency Virus," *Pediatrics* 79(3):466-71, March 1987.

Blanchet, Kevin D. *AIDS: A Health Care Management Response.* Rockville, Md.: Aspen Systems, 1988.

Hughes, R.B., and Bailey, F.K. "Aids From a School Health Perspective," *Pediatric Nursing* 13(3):155-56, June 1987.

Klug, R.M. "Children with AIDS, Part 2" *AJN* 86(10):1126-32, October 1987.

Loveman, A., et al. "AIDS in Pregnancy," *JOGNN* 15(2):91-93, March/April 1986.

Whaley, L.F., and Wong, D.L. *Nursing Care of Infants and Children,* 3rd ed. St. Louis: C.V. Mosby Co, 1987.

Chapter 7

Scipien, G., et al. *Comprehensive Pediatric Nursing,* 3rd ed. New York: McGraw-Hill Book Co., 1986.

Whaley, L., and Wong, D. *Essentials of Pediatric Nursing,* 3rd ed., St. Louis: C.V. Mosby Co., 1987.

Chapter 8

Adams, D. "Children with Ostomies: Comprehensive Care Planning," *Pediatric Nursing* 12(6):429-33, November/December 1986.

Brunner, L., and Suddarth, D. *Lippincott Manual of Nursing Practice,"* 4th ed. Philadelphia: J.B. Lippincott Co., 1986.

Candy, C.E. "Recent Advances in the Care of Children with Acute Diarrhea: Giving Responsibility to the Nurse and Parents," *Journal of Advanced Nursing* 12(1):95-99, January 1987.

Harris, J. "Pediatric Abdominal Assessment," *Pediatric Nursing* 12(5): 355-62, September/October 1986.

Khatib, H. "Acute Gastroenteritis in Infants," *Nursing Times* 82(17): 31-32, April 23-29, 1986.

Marlow, D., and Redding, B. *Textbook of Pediatric Nursing,* 6th ed. Philadelphia: W.B. Saunders Co., 1988.

Pate, C. "Care of the Family Following the Birth of a Child with a Cleft Lip and/or Palate," *Neonatal Network* 5(6):30-37, June 1987.

Scipien, G., et al. *Comprehensive Pediatric Nursing,* 3rd ed. New York: McGraw-Hill Book Co., 1986.

Chapter 9

Barbarin, O., and Chesler, M. "The Medical Context of Parental Coping with Childhood Cancer," *American Journal of Community Psychology* 14(2):221-35, April 1986.

Cohen, D.G., et al. "Growing Up Differently: An Adolescent's Perspective," *Seminars in Oncology Nursing* 2(2):84-89, May 1986.

Hockenberry, M.J., and Coody, D.K. *Pediatric Oncology and Hematology: Perspectives on Care.* St. Louis: C.V. Mosby Co., 1986.

Jennings, C. "Children's Understanding of Death and Dying," *Focus on Critical Care* 13(1):41-45, February 1986.

Landier, W.C., et al. "How to Administer Blood Components to Children," *Journal of Maternal-Child Nursing* 12:178-84, May/June 1987.

Maul-Mellott, S.K., and Adams, J.N. *Childhood Cancer: A Nursing Overview.* Boston: Jones & Bartlett Publishers, 1987.

Neuberger, Julia. "A Crying Shame...Dying Patients Like Their Nurses to Share Their Anger and Their Grief," *Nursing Times* 82(12):22, March 19-25, 1986.

Reynolds, E.A., and Ramenofsky, M.L. "The Emotional Impact of Trauma on Toddlers," *MCN* 13(2):106-09, March/April 1988.

Trouy, M., and Ward-Larson, R. "Sibling Grief," *Neonatal Network* 5(4):35-40, February 1987.

Walker, K.L. "I Really Don't Know What to Say...Dealing with Bereaved Family Members," *Emergency Medical Services* 16(1):42-43, January/February 1987.

Whaley, L.F., and Wong, D.L., eds. *Nursing Care of Infants and Children,* 4th ed. St. Louis: Mosby-Year Book, 1991.

Chapter 10

Deering, C.G. "Developing a Therapeutic Alliance with the Anorexia Nervosa Client," *Journal of Psychosocial Nursing* 25(3):10-17, 37, March 1987.

Muscari, M. "Identification and Management of the Early Anorectic Child," *Journal of Pediatric Health Care* 1(4):196-203, July/August 1987.

Muscari, M. "Adolescent Suicide Attempts by Acetaminophen Ingestion," *MCN* 12(1):32-35, January/February 1987.

Spitz, H.I., and Rosecan, J.S., eds. *Cocaine Abuse: New Directions in Treatment and Research.* New York: Brunner-Mazel, 1987.

Valente, S.M. "Assessing Suicide Risk in the School-Age Child," *Journal of Pediatric Health Care* 1(1):14-20, January/February 1987.

Washton, A.M., and Gold, M.S., eds. *Cocaine: A Clinician's Handbook.* New York: Guilford Press, 1987.

Chapter 11

American Diabetes Association. "Office Guide to Diagnosis and Classification of Diabetes Mellitus and Other Categories of Glucose Intolerance," *Diabetes Care* 13(Supp. 1):3-4, January 1990.

Boswell, E.J. "Selecting Teaching Strategies to Promote Patient Adherence," *Diabetes Education* 13(4):410-12, Fall 1987.

Drass, J., et al. "Reviewing Diabetes," *Nursing90* 20(4):120-22, 124, April 1990.

Marlow, D., and Redding, B. *Textbook of Pediatric Nursing,* 6th ed. Philadelphia: W.B. Saunders Co., 1988.

Scipien, G., et al. *Comprehensive Pediatric Nursing,* 3rd ed. New York: McGraw-Hill Book Co., 1986.

Whaley, L., and Wong, D. *Nursing Care of Infants and Children.* St. Louis: C.V. Mosby Co., 1987.

Chapter 12

Klaus, M.H., and Fanaroff, A.A. *Care of the High-Risk Neonate,* 3rd ed. Philadelphia: W.B. Saunders Co., 1986.

Korones, S. *High-Risk Newborn Infants: The Basis for Intensive Nursing Care,* 4th ed. St. Louis: C.V. Mosby Co., 1986.

Rudolph, A.M., and Hoffman, J.I.E. *Pediatrics,* 18th ed. Norwalk, Conn.: Appleton & Lange, 1987.

Whaley, L.F., and Wong, D.L. *Nursing Care of Infants and Children.* St. Louis: C.V. Mosby Co., 1987.

Chapter 13

Fisk, R. "Management of the Pediatric Cardiovascular Patient after Surgery," *Critical Care Quarterly* 9(2):75-82, September 1986.

Girlando, R.M., et al. "Coarctation of the Aorta," *Critical Care Nurse* 8(1):38-50, January/February 1988.

Higgins, S., and Kashani, I. "The Cyanotic Child: Heart Defects and Parental Learning Needs," *MCN* 11(4):259-62, July/August 1986.

Horner, M.M., et al. "How Parents of Children with Chronic Conditions Perceive Their Own Needs," *MCN* 12(1):40-43, January/February 1987.

Joffe, M. "Pediatric Digoxin Administration," *Dimensions of Critical Care Nursing* 6(3):136-46, May/June 1987.

Kashani, I., and Higgins, S. "Counseling Strategies for Families of Children with Heart Disease," *Pediatric Nursing* 12(1):38-40, January/February 1986.

Lawrence, P.A., and Wieczorek, B.H. "Congenital Valvular Heart Disease," *Journal of Cardiovascular Nursing* 1(3):18-25, May, 1987.

Malinowski, P., and Yablonski, C. "Congenital Heart Disease in Infants: Nursing Assessment," *Critical Care Quarterly* 9(2):6-23, September 1986.

Pilichi, L.M. "Supporting the Parents When the Child Requires Intensive Care," *Focus on Critical Care* 15(2):34-38, April 1988.

Pillitteri, A. *Child Health Nursing,* 3rd ed. Boston: Little, Brown & Co., 1987.

Potter, P.A., and Perry, A.G. *Fundamentals of Nursing,* 2nd ed. St. Louis: Mosby Year-Book, 1989.

Runton, N. "Congenital Cardiac Anomalies: A Reference Guide for Nurses," *Journal of Cardiovascular Nursing* 2(3):56-70, May 1988.

Servonsky, J., and Opec, S. *Nursing Management of Children.* Jones & Barlett Publishers, 1987.

Slota, M.C. "Assessment of Systemic Perfusion in the Child," *Critical Care Nursing* 7(4):68-73, July/August 1987.

Smith, M., et al. *Child and Family: Concepts of Nursing Practice,* 2nd ed. New York: McGraw-Hill Book Co., 1987.

Whaley, L.F., and and Wong, D.L. *Nursing Care of Infants and Children,* 3rd ed. St. Louis: C.V. Mosby Co., 1987.

Chapter 14
Greenberg, C.S., ed. *Nursing Care Planning Guides for Children.* Baltimore: Williams & Wilkins Co., 1988.

Luckmann, J., and Sorensen, K. *Medical-Surgical Nursing: A Psychophysiologic Approach,* 3rd ed. Philadelphia: W.B. Saunders Co., 1987.

Marlow, D., and Redding, B. *Textbook of Pediatric Nursing,* 6th ed. Philadelphia: W.B. Saunders Co., 1988.

Mott, S., et al. *Nursing Care of Children and Families: A Holistic Approach,* 2nd ed. Redwood City, Calif.: Addison Wesley Publishing Co., 1990.

Whaley, L., and Wong, D. *Nursing Care of Infants and Children.* St. Louis: C.V. Mosby Co., 1987.

Wong, D., and Whaley, L. *Clinical Manual of Pediatric Nursing,* 3rd ed. St. Louis: Mosby Year-Book, 1990.

Yanko, J.R. "Seizures and What They Mean for Your Patient," *Nursing87* 17(9):32C, 32F, September 1987.

Chapter 15
Cohen, A. "Management of Iron Overload in the Pediatric Patient," *Hematology/Oncology Clinics of North America* 1(3):521-44, September 1987.

Eaton, W., and Hofrichter, J. "Hemoglobin S. Gelation and Sickle Cell Disease," *Blood* 70(5):1245-66, November 1987.

Kempe, C. *Current Pediatric Diagnosis and Treatment,* 9th ed. Norwalk, Conn.: Appleton & Lange, 1987.

Gaston, M.H., et al. "Prophylaxis with Oral Penicillin in Children with Sickle Cell Anemia," *New England Journal of Medicine* 314(25):1593-99, June 19, 1986.

Hayes, J., et al. "Managing PKU: An Update," *MCN* 12(2):119-23, March/April 1987.

Hollenberg, J.P., et al. "Cost-Effectiveness of Splenectomy Versus Intravenous Gamma Globulin in Treatment of Chronic Immune Thrombocytopenic Purpura in Childhood," *Journal of Pediatrics* 112(4):530-39, April 1988.

Kelting, S., and Johnson, C. "Erythropoiesis and Neonatal Blood Transfusions," *MCN* 12(3):172-77, June 1987.

Moore, K. *The Developing Human,* 4th ed. Philadelphia: W.B. Saunders Co., 1988.

Ohene-Frempong, K., et al. "Thalassemia Syndromes: Recent Advances," *Hematology/Oncolocy Clinics of North America* 1(3):503-19, September 1987.

Pelligra, S.J. "Hemophilia: Pathophysiology and Musculoskeletal Complications," *Southern Medical Journal* 80(9):1148-52, September 1987.

Withers, J., and Bradshaw, E. "Preventive Neonatal Hepatitis-B Infection," *MCN* 11(4):270-272, July/August 1986.

Chapter 16

Friedland, G.H., and Klein, R.S. "Transmission of the Human Immunodeficiency Virus," *New England Journal of Medicine* 317(18):1125-35, October 29, 1987.

McCray, E., and Martone, W.J. "Preventing HIV Exposure Among Patients and Staff," *AIDS Patient Care* 1(2):32-34, September 1987.

Sachs, B., et al. "Acquired Immunodeficiency Syndrome: Suggested Protocol for Counseling and Screening in Pregnancy," *Obstetrics & Gynecology* 70(3 Part 1):408-11, September 1987.

Whaley, L.F., and Wong, D.L. *Nursing Care of Infants and Children,* 3rd ed. St. Louis: C.V. Mosby Co., 1987.

White, K. "Special Precautions for Managing Pediatric AIDS," *AIDS Patient Care* 1(2):10-12, September 1987.

Index

Temperature
  axillary, 129, 139, 249, 257
  rectal, 28, 41
Temper tantrums, 6-7, 19, 66
Testes
  enlargement of, 4
  undescended, 77, 85
Testosterone, 220
Tetracycline, 81, 89
Tetralogy of Fallot, 245-248, 254, 256,
    295, 297, 320, 322
Theophylline, 231, 242
Throat culture, 56, 68, 119, 126
Thrombocytopenia, 44
Thrombosis, 247, 256
Thyroid, assessment of, 56, 69
Thyroid function studies, 172, 184
Thyroxine, 212, 219
Tissue hypoxia, 296, 322
Toddlers
  growth in, 6, 19
  pain symptoms of, 157, 168
  play and, 3, 15
  psychosocial development of, 20
  toilet training of, 3, 4, 16, 303,
    329-330
Toe clubbing, 247, 256
Toe pointing, 267, 278
Tofranil, 101, 113
Toilet training, 3, 4, 16, 303, 329-330
Tongue blade, 230, 241
Tonic neck reflex, 52, 63, 299, 324
Tonsillectomy, 229-230, 240-242, 302,
    328
Total parenteral nutrition (TPN), 31, 44,
    175, 188, 315, 342-343
Toys, age-appropriate, 3, 15
TPN tubing, 31, 44
Tracheoesophageal fistula, 311-312, 338-
    339
Tracheostomy set, 229, 240
Transfusion, 30, 43, 55, 67
Trazodone, 101, 113
Tricuspid atresia, 249, 257-258
Trisomy 21, 28, 40
Twins, 28, 40
Twitching, 310, 337
Tylenol, 135, 146
Tyrosine, 310, 337

U

Umbilical cord, 29, 41-42
Umbilical vein, 131, 141
Universal precautions, 121, 127, 314, 342
Urinary tract infection, 81, 89, 149, 159
Urine test, 214, 221

V

Vagus, stimulation of, 102, 114-115
Vagina, discharge from, 80, 88
Varicella, 56, 68, 261, 272-273
Vascular system, access to, 131
Vasodilators, 249, 258
Venous access device, 173, 186
Ventilation, 223, 234
  mechanical, 224, 236
Ventricular septal defect, 245, 295, 320
Vibration, 224, 235
Vincristine, 171, 177, 183, 189
Virus, 262, 274
Vision screening, 8, 20
Visual stimulation, 298, 323-324
Vital signs, 247, 255
Vitamin A & D ointment, 174, 187
Vitamin A-rich foods, 93, 105
Voice, muffling of, 229, 240
Voice disorder, 17, 18
Vomiting, 136, 147, 149, 159
  self-induced, 100-101, 112

W

Walking, 95, 107
Weight gain, infants and, 98, 110, 225,
    236
Weight loss, 173, 186-186
  in anorexic patient, 102
  in cancer patient, 172, 184
  in diabetic patient, 211, 217, 304, 331
  in neonate, 34, 47
  program for, 95, 107-108
Western blot, 313, 340
Whey, 118, 124
White blood cell count, 334
Wilm's tumor, 177, 189

XYZ